Shirley Plant

Finally... Food I Can Eat!

Balboa Press books may be ordered through booksellers or by contacting:

Balboa Press
A Division of Hay House
1663 Liberty Drive
Bloomington, IN 47403
www.balboapress.com
1-(877) 407-4847

Because of the dynamic nature of the Internet, any web addresses or links contained in this book may have changed since publication and may no longer be valid. The views expressed in this work are solely those of the author and do not necessarily reflect the views of the publisher, and the publisher hereby disclaims any responsibility for them.

Legal Disclaimer
The information contained in this cookbook is not intended to replace the advice or treatments offered by your physician. If you suspect you have allergies or food intolerances, please seek medical advice. If your allergies are severe or life threatening, be sure to check all ingredients carefully to ensure none of them contain food allergens before cooking. No promises or warranties, expressed or implied, as to the appropriateness of any food or recipes for a particular person's diet are made by this book. No liability will be assumed by anyone affiliated with the writing, production, or distribution of this book for any damages arising from the preparation or consumption of the foods described herein, whether such losses are special, incidental, consequential, or otherwise. The reader accepts sole responsibility for the use of the information contained in this book.

The author of this book does not dispense medical advice or prescribe the use of any technique as a form of treatment for physical, emotional, or medical problems without the advice of a physician, either directly or indirectly. The intent of the author is only to offer information of a general nature to help you in your quest for emotional and spiritual well-being. In the event you use any of the information in this book for yourself, which is your constitutional right, the author and the publisher assume no responsibility for your actions.

ISBN: 978-1-4525-6110-3 (e)
ISBN: 978-1-4525-6109-7 (sc)

Library of Congress Control Number: 2012920157

Printed in the United States of America

Balboa Press rev. date: 11/5/2012

Shirley Plant

Finally... Food I Can Eat!

A dietary guide and cookbook featuring tasty non-vegetarian and
vegetarian recipes for people with food allergies and food intolerances.

BALBOA
PRESS
A DIVISION OF HAY HOUSE

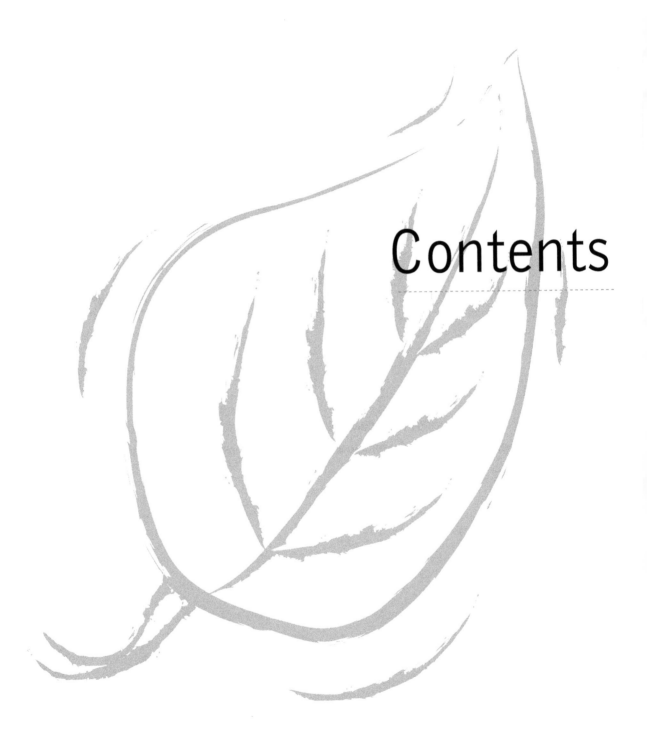

Contents

Introduction
7

About this Cookbook
10

About Allergies and Intolerances
13

A Quick Guide to Natural Food Chemicals
19

Food Additives
23

Substitutes for Common Foods
28

Basic Food Combining
41

Helpful Hints to the Cook
43

Breakfast and Juices
46

Main Dishes and Lunches
64

Soups
98

Salads and Dressings
114

Snacks and Spreads
146

Desserts
164

Food Families
204

Rotation Diet
219

Allergen Avoidance Index
225

Metric Conversion
236

Sunshine Cake

Fill a measure full of sunshine,

Some crumbs of comfort too;

Then mix them well with loving thoughts

And words both kind and true.

Let them quickly rise with action

To deeds of golden hue,

And you'll have a cake worth eating

When baking time is through.

Yes, you'll have a life worth living

And a cure for every ache

If you add all your family

You'll feast on "Sunshine Cake."

Introduction

- Some, it is said, like to cook. Others cannot be bothered and prefer to eat out.

For those of us who suffer from food allergies and food intolerances, it is difficult at times to make the simplest of meals, let alone eat out at a restaurant. We are the ones who are allergic to dairy, wheat, yeast, eggs, corn, sugar, and soy; and the list goes on. Newly diagnosed with these food allergies can leave you at a loss as to what to eat and how to prepare it. So if you have just discovered that you have food allergies, or food intolerances, or you know someone who is struggling with what to eat because of diet limitations, then here is the cookbook for you! I have heard people cry, "There is nothing left to eat. What can I eat now?" Or "How do I cook millet or quinoa? I have never even heard of them." FINALLY... FOOD I CAN EAT! is a cookbook for allergy sufferers, those who need to rotate their foods, and health-conscious individuals. Let FINALLY... FOOD I CAN EAT! be your guide to a simpler, tastier life. This cookbook will enable people who suffer from food allergies, food intolerances, celiac disease, and those looking for low-sugar, low-cholesterol and heart-smart diets to cook easy, healthy meals that are free of the foods that can make them feel sick or make their conditions worse. These recipes can also offer variety to those who are limited to eating only a few foods and will even appeal to picky eaters. They are also designed to save you time and energy. By introducing new foods into your diet, your general health and well-being may improve, too! These recipes will help you find alternatives to what you have been eating and at the same time bring you hope that you can eat yummy foods again. I passionately believe that anyone can make themselves something tasty to eat, even if dealing with food allergies and intolerances. It may not look as fluffy as it did when you baked with eggs and white flour, but after all, it simply is food. Cooking is a whole lot easier than many of us think, and introducing new foods should not make it any harder. The recipes in this book are simple. There is no flashy presentation, which doesn't mean they won't satisfy and please. Some of these recipes are very different and use ingredients like hemp or teff. Others are like an old friend: they comfort us, like beef stew and shepherd's pie. Some call for a handful of parsley while others have exact measurements as needed. I urge you to be brave and use herbs and spices that tantalize and please you. The options are yours. That is what is so wonderful about cooking.

I dedicate this book to my mother, Mary Plant, whom I love and miss every day. Thanks for teaching me to cook, Mum. To my family and Charlie, who is always there for me, and to all those who suffer daily with food allergies, intolerances, and sensitivities.

I wish to thank my family and friends for their love and support. Eric, Vivianne, Carolyn, Steve, Sophia, David, thanks for taste testing. A special thanks to my friend Greg Coleman, who without fail or complaint tasted most of these recipes. To Shanny, Lucie, and the students at La Cité Collégiale who helped with design work.

About this
Cookbook

The idea of this cookbook came to me while I was living in Sydney, Australia. Whether in Ottawa, Canada, or Sydney, Australia, I had difficulty in finding a cookbook that had recipes for food that I could eat. I suffer from food intolerances and allergies, and every time I wanted to make something, I had to substitute at least three or four food items in the recipe. As you can guess, they were time-consuming to make, and recipes did not turn out. Since I also suffer from Chronic Fatigue Syndrome, I did not have the energy to keep trying the recipe again and again until I got it right. It certainly is no fun when you cannot eat your own birthday cake because you are allergic to all its ingredients, or are not able to partake of the Christmastime hors d'oeuvres. After a few years of eating the same dry rice cakes and muffins, I decided to develop some of my own recipes by substituting foods that I could eat into my favourite recipes. I used spelt flour instead of whole wheat flour, flaxseeds instead of eggs, rice milk instead of regular milk, kamut or quinoa pasta, and fruit or stevia to sweeten. Before I knew it, I had recipes that were easy to make, tasted good, and were within the confines of my allergies.

Over the years, friends who had food allergies started asking me for my recipes, as did others who wanted to just eat well or who wanted to introduce new foods into their diet. Friends whose children were diagnosed with food allergies started asking me what kind of cookies I ate, and what could they possibly use instead of wheat, milk, and eggs? Well, I am pleased to say all these questions are answered in this cookbook.

Remember, it may take you awhile to become adjusted to some of these new foods. It certainly did for me, but now I am content and love foods like teff, millet, carob, hemp, and rice milk. I also know that I am eating different foods and rotating them, which is much healthier than eating the same processed bread and sugar-filled snack day after day. Because every individual has different food intolerances and restrictions, I have written a chapter on how to substitute foods specifically for you (see page 28). This will help you to rotate foods throughout your diet. You will also find a list of food chemicals that occur naturally in foods that can cause many people problems with their health. Also noted are some helpful hints to assist you with adapting to your new foods. Each of us is unique in how our body responds to different foods. We all live in different climates and geographical locations, so one diet will not necessarily be appropriate for everyone. Some foods are not available in certain parts of the world. You might ask, what is the right diet for me? One that is practical, easy to stay on, eliminates the foods that are bothering you, and makes you feel better. Taking time to prepare healthy meals = a healthy body, mind, and spirit. Fortunately, we now have wonderful health food stores and supermarkets that feature organic produce and a wider variety of foods. Stores now carry wheat-free/yeast-free breads, tofu, rice milk, spelt pastas, and other grains that are healthy, tasty, and easy to prepare. If you could prepare easy, healthy, delicious meals for yourself and your family, with the knowledge that they did not contain colourings, chemical additives, preservatives, and refined sugars, and that it would not take you all day to cook them, would you be interested? I think most people would, but with our busy schedules, time and energy is not an easy thing to come by. Many recipes take time and energy to make, and when you have food allergies you need to substitute everything in your current cookbook; this may make you decide to order take-out or skimp on your meals. You buy prepackaged meals that have preservatives, additives, and other ingredients in them that will continue to make you feel unwell.

Many people these days are experiencing health problems that are due to poor nutrition. Now I am sure that most of you think you are eating a healthful, balanced diet, but in fact you are probably not. A lot of health issues such as hypertension, depression, obesity, heart disease, arthritis, allergies, diabetes, and gastrointestinal and skin disorders stem from poor nutrition. Studies show that most North Americans feel that they are obtaining an adequate diet based on their knowledge of nutrition. We are also hounded by advertising of unhealthy foods every day on television and radio, but because they are quick and easy and the food and drug companies endorse them, we believe they are healthy.

Perhaps if we promoted healthier diets and fewer fast foods we would see an increase in healthier people and fewer chronic disorders. Our environment has changed, and we now overprocess our foods and produce our foods much more quickly than ever before. We are able to eat foods in the winter season that years ago we would never get until the summer growing season was upon us. Our habits have changed, our lives are much more fast-paced, and we live in a world full of chemicals. Should we supplement our diets with synthetic vitamins, or are we getting our recommended daily allowances needed for optimal health through our food? So what is the answer, you might ask?

I believe that you should start by being more aware of what you are putting into your body. Try to broaden your diet so that you are not eating the same foods all the time. It is recognized that overindulgence of the same foods is one of the causes of food intolerance. Keep in mind that you are sometimes selecting foods that have been heavily processed, and many of them have no nutritional value. Begin to read labels, and when you have the choice, choose natural foods closest to what Mother Nature intended for us to eat.

About Allergies
and Intolerances

- What is the difference between food allergy and food intolerance?
- Do certain foods upset you after you have eaten them?
- Do you know someone who reacts to certain foods?

This part of the book will tell you about intolerances and allergies.

Food Allergies and Intolerances

Definitions

Allergy refers to a response of the immune system. It involves immunological processes similar to (but not exactly the same as) those that fight and reject an agent that can cause diseases, such as a pathogenic (disease-causing) micro-organism.

Hypersensitivity is the term scientists use to describe the immunological process that results in allergy. The terms allergic reaction and hypersensitivity reaction are often used interchangeably.

Food intolerance refers to a reaction that does not involve the immune system. It is caused by a problem in the way the body processes the food or food additive. The term food intolerance is not interchangeable with either food allergy or hypersensitivity.

Food sensitivity is a rather non-specific term that refers to a person's reacting adversely to a food or component of the food when it is not clear whether the reaction is due to allergy or intolerance. The term food sensitivity is therefore interchangeable with either food allergy or food intolerance, but it does not give any indication of the reason for a person's symptoms.

Food sensitivities can affect any organ system in the body. Fatigue, anxiety, depression, insomnia, obesity, ear infections, post-nasal drip, irritable bowel syndrome, diarrhea, Crohn's disease, high blood pressure, eczema, hives, muscle aches, headaches, migraines, and asthma are some of the symptoms due to food allergy.

Allergy Types

Our immune system can produce symptoms simply as a result of our ingesting food; this is known as a food allergy. Food allergies are classified into four types:

- I anaphylactic
- II cytotoxic
- III antigen-antibody complexes
- IV delayed hypersensitivity

There are two types of allergic reaction: fixed and cyclic. Fixed reactions are IgE-mediated and are easily recognized. If you eat a particular food and immediately get sick or break out, you know what food is triggering the reaction, especially if it happens every time you eat that specific food. Cyclic or delayed food allergy is hard to detect. Sometimes the reaction can be delayed and symptoms appear hours or days later. It is estimated that only five percent of food allergy is immediate and ninety-five percent is delayed.[1]

Type I Reactions

Anaphylaxis is usually IgE-mediated. In this instance, the body manufactures an antibody when a foreign substance (an antigen) gains access to the intestines, lungs, or skin.

An anaphylactic reaction is fixed and can vary from mild to fatal, but usually appears within minutes of ingestion of the food. It can affect the respiratory tract (bronchial obstruction, wheezing), the gastrointestinal tract (nausea, vomiting, bloating, or diarrhea), the cardiovascular system (hypotension and shock), and the skin (hives). Sensitivity to the food usually persists for more than two years, even after the food is removed from the diet; therefore, the only treatment for this is elimination of the offending food.

Type II and Type III Reactions

Cytotoxic reactions (type II) involve IgG- or IgM-mediated responses and are cyclic in nature. IgG and IgM are antibodies that are made to defend our immune system. Unlike a fixed food allergy, a cyclic allergy is exposure-dependent. Therefore, the more frequently a sensitive food is ingested, the greater the IgG reaction, which leads to increased sensitivity. Treatment for this type of allergy is to eliminate the food for six months, then reintroduce it to the diet, but not eat it every day. The reason for eliminating the food for six months is so the IgG falls to a low level. When the food is reintroduced, there will be a slight elevation of IgG, but limited exposure will keep the IgG level low, therefore not producing allergic symptoms.

Doctors suggest a rotation diet in which the suspected food is eaten only every four days. Infrequent exposure to this food ensures that IgG reactions will not become elevated and reactive symptoms high. Type III reactions are when antigen-antibody complexes are formed in the blood. Symptoms are not always immediate and can be delayed, therefore not always relating to food ingestion. Like type II, they are difficult to to diagnose.

Type IV Reactions

These are cell-mediated immune reactions, which are triggered by the interaction between actively sensitized lymphocytes and specific antigens. These types of cyclic reactions can be the most difficult to diagnose, as the T-cell effect develops twenty-four to seventy-two hours after the ingestion of the antigen, so it is difficult to say which food is causing the reaction.

Skin tests and IgE Rast tests will not detect these, so doctors often tell people that they do not have food allergies when in fact they do.

Notes

1   Boyles, J.H. Jr., "Introduction to food allergy: history and characteristics," In: Krause, H.F., ed., Otolaryngic Allergy and Immunology (Philadelphia: WB Saunders, 1989), 218.

Definitions reprinted with permission from *Dealing With Food Allergies,* by Janice Vickerstaff Joneja, © 2003, Bull Publishing Company.

There are many ways of testing for allergies. Listed below are a few of these allergy testing techniques.

One test to help detect food allergies is the Individual Challenge Feeding Test. This test is based on reaction to two closely spaced feedings of a specific food.

- Each food tested must be avoided for at least 4 days, but no more than 10 days prior to testing

- Check your pulse before you eat the food in question

- Ingest a specific food and nothing else

- Test your pulse very 20, 40 and 60 minutes after eating

If the pulse rate has increased without symptoms a sensitivity is probable. An increased pulse rate with symptoms indicates a sensitivity.

- One hour later ingest the same food

- Observe pulse rate and symptoms for 30 minutes

If no reaction occurs, include test food with your evening meal and watch for delayed symptoms at night.

Other allergy tests include: The Standard Scratch or Prick Test. This is when an area of skin, usually the upper arm or back, is pricked with a needle and a drop of antigen is placed where it can be absorbed into the skin. If the person is sensitive to the antigen, a bump or red area will form on the skin and the allergy will be noted. If the person has low IgE levels, many times a skin reaction will not occur. Or if the person only has food intolerances, which indicates an IgG response, or a delayed allergy, this type of testing will be of no benefit.

Blood Allergy Testing: Blood allergy tests are available through various labs for allergy testing, and can test for both IgE and IgG mediated responses.

Sublingual Provocative Testing: A baseline pulse rate is taken before testing begins. The test antigen is then placed under the tongue of the patient and is held there for one minute. This helps with faster absorption into the bloodstream. After five minutes, the pulse is measured and compared with the first baseline pulse. Also noted are any symptoms in the patient. If there are any changes observed, a positive is said to have occurred and then either stronger or weaker dilutions of the same antigen are administered until the patient's pulse is back to the baseline and symptoms have disappeared.

Vega Test or Electrodermal Testing: This is a popular method of allergy testing in both Europe and North America. It is based on the concept that slight changes in the electrical impedance of a person's skin occur when an allergen is placed on an electrical circuit. The patient holds an electrode in his/her hand that is connected by circuit to a probe held by the practitioner. The practitioner places an allergen in the holder on the circuit and then touches the probe to an acupuncture point on the patient's skin. The greater the sensitivity of the patient to the allergen, the higher the reading on the galvanometer. There are no scientific studies to confirm this type of testing at this time.

Other forms of allergy tests are Applied Kinesiology or Muscle Strength testing. Many of these tests are based on a holistic approach and are sometimes viewed by the medical community as not conclusive. Once again there is no scientific proof to support these tests.

Common food allergies

Common food allergies are wheat, egg, milk, shellfish, and peanuts. These allergies can cause swelling, itching, cramps, and diarrhea, and may even cause ana-phylactic shock or fatigue. Some allergic responses are immediate, like wheezing or itchy eyes, but some reactions can be delayed, making it difficult to distinguish the cause. Delayed reactions may include joint aches, eczema, migraine, diarrhea, hyperactivity, fatigue, and depression.

Are you allergic?

Some people have difficulty in determining if they are allergic, as many of the symptoms are masked or hidden. When you eat a food often, such as milk, you may constantly have a stuffy nose but will not attribute it to the milk that you drink three times a day. Sometimes when the milk is removed, a stuffy nose can get worse before it gets better. This is called the withdrawal response and it is like kicking the habit.

Children with food allergies may look tired and can have dark circles under their eyes. They tend to have earaches or ear infections. They may have difficulty concentrating in school and may be irritable. The good news is that most of these symptoms disappear when the allergic food is eliminated.

People crave the very foods to which they are allergic, so a good way to find out what you are allergic to is to ask yourself what food is it that you would not be able to live without?

The onslaught of allergies on the body can result in a lowered immune system, and illness can follow, so it is very important to find out what you are allergic to and address this problem.

Rotation diet

A rotation diet is a way to eat a wide range of different foods and is highly recommended when you have found out that you are allergic or food intolerant. It is organized in such a manner that you do not eat the same foods day after day. When you become allergic, and are told to omit a certain food, you might simply replace it with another food that is similar or from the same food family (see page 205). If you eat that new food daily, you run the risk of becoming allergic or intolerant to it as well.

There are different types of rotation diets. The most common is a four-day rotation diet. What this means is that any food will be eaten only once in four days and avoided for the rest of the week. When you start your rotation diet, you will avoid all the foods that your doctor has advised. Once you start this, you may notice that you begin to feel better. Be careful not to cheat at this time, as you want to give your system a chance to benefit from your rotation diet. If you do cheat and you feel unwell, you will know right away that the food in question is one you should avoid for a period of time. Some doctors recommend that you stay on your rotation diet for at least three months. For help with planning out your rotation diet, see a dietitian, nutritionist, or naturopathic doctor, or e-mail me, Shirley Plant, info@deliciousalternatives.com, Web site www.deliciousalternatives.com, as I consult and plan weekly menus for people newly diagnosed with food allergies.

For a sample rotation diet, please see page 220.

A Quick Guide to
Natural Food Chemicals

Introduction

Chemicals are found everywhere. We find them in nature as well as in our food. Sometimes they are beneficial and sometimes they are poisonous. These days, many people seem to be sensitive to natural chemicals that are found in our foods and environment.

Reactions to food chemicals are sometimes inherited, but anyone can develop symptoms at any age. Natural chemicals can pose just as many problems to people as artificial chemicals used as food additives. Usually, the tastier the food, the more likely it is to contain natural or artificial chemicals.

Phenols are chemicals found in foods that some people have difficulty processing. These chemicals build up to levels in the body that can affect them physically. Salicylate, a natural chemical and subgroup of phenol, can cause similar symptoms and is made by many food plants. It is chemically related to aspirin, which is a derivative of salicylic acid. Although salicylates are found in wholesome foods, some individuals have difficulty tolerating them even in small amounts. The reaction to a natural salicylate can be as severe as that to synthetic additives if a person is highly sensitive.

Some symptoms of salicylate sensitivity are: asthma, hives, stomach upset, dark circles under the eyes, diarrhea, hyperactivity, headache, and wheezing.

What follows is a quick guide to some of the more important natural chemicals and a list of foods that are high and low in salicylates.

You may wish to eliminate, or at least reduce, these foods to prevent overload and reactions. After omitting these foods, see if you are starting to feel a bit better. Then, after a few weeks, take a challenge test and try one of the omitted foods to see if it still bothers you. Remember, though, that symptoms might not recur for several days, because the effect could be cumulative.

Before you try to tackle these challenges yourself, you should seek medical attention. Your doctor might suggest allergy testing, but remember that normal allergy testing will not tell you if you are sensitive to certain foods—only that you are allergic to them. So in fact you may still be feeling poorly even after you realize you are allergic to certain foods and have eliminated them from your diet. It is best to see an environmental doctor, naturopath, or nutritionist who can help you with an elimination diet to see if you are, in fact, food sensitive as well.

Some Common Natural Chemicals

Amines	Amines come from the breakdown of protein. They are found in fermented products like cheese, wines, chocolate, bananas, avocados, and tomatoes. Amine levels can rise when grilling or browning meat.
MSG	Monosodium glutamate—or MSG—is found naturally in some foods. Foods rich in natural MSG are tomatoes, mushrooms, and cheeses. MSG is often used to enhance the flavour of soups, sauces, snack foods, and Chinese food. Some items such as canned tuna might contain MSG, but it is sometimes difficult to identify. Manufacturers may use such names as sodium caseinate, hydrolyzed yeast, hydrolyzed vegetable protein, yeast extract, natural flavouring, or "other spices."
Salicylates	Salicylates are a family of plant chemicals. They are found naturally in fruits, vegetables, nuts, spices, tea, coffee, perfumes, flavourings, and medications. Aspirin is a member of the salicylate family. Salicylate levels are higher in unripe fruits and decrease with ripening. Listed below are foods and their salicylate levels.

Very high—avoid

> raisins, prunes

> aniseed, cayenne, celery powder, cinnamon, curry, dill, Chinese five spices, garum masala, mace, mustard, oregano, paprika, rosemary, sage, tarragon, turmeric, thyme, Worcester sauce

High—avoid

> apples (sharp, such as Granny Smith), berries, citrus fruits, currants, dried fruits, figs, guavas, grapes, kiwi fruit, pineapple

> broccoli, chicory, endive, gherkins, mushrooms, peppers, radishes, watercress

> allspice, bay leaves, chili, cloves, ginger, mint, nutmeg, black pepper, pickles

> almonds, pistachios, macadamia nuts, pine nuts

> honey, licorice, peppermint, chewing gum

> black tea, rum, port, Tia Maria, Benedictine, Drambuie

Moderate—eat occasionally

> apricots, dates, lychee, peaches, plums

> asparagus, avocados, cucumbers, cauliflowers, onions, squash, tomatoes (tinned)
> white pepper
> Brazil nuts, walnuts
> corn flour
> coffee (instant), rose hip tea, beer, cider, sherry, red and white wine

Low—eat freely

> apples (not sharp), bananas, mangoes, passion fruit, pawpaw, pears (peeled), persimmons, papayas, pomegranates, rhubarb
> chickpeas, dried beans, French beans, bean sprouts, beetroot, cabbage, carrots, celery, leeks, lentils, lettuce, peas, split peas, potatoes, rutabaga, shallots, spinach, sweet corn, tomatoes (fresh and juice), turnips
> coriander leaves, garlic, fresh parsley, saffron, soy sauce, Tabasco sauce, Tandoori powder, vinegar (malt)
> cashews, dried coconut, hazelnuts, peanuts, pecans, poppy seeds, sesame seeds, sunflower seeds
> all cereals except corn flour
> all meats, fish, shellfish, milk, cheese
> most herbal teas, decaffeinated black tea, brandy, gin, vodka, whisky

Food
Additives

Approximately eighty percent of the foods we consume today are refined and chemically altered. Food additives are not natural flavouring, spices, or seasonings. The FDA in the United States allows more than 15,000 food and chemical additives in our food supply. The average American consumes 10-15 pounds of salt and additives per year. Food additives make the food more pleasing to the eyes and also prevent some foods from spoiling and increases their shelf life, but at what cost? Food additives can pose problems as well. Preservatives are used these days to keep food fresh longer, and colourings are used to make food look more attractive to the consumer.

Here is a quick guide to the "nasties" on your grocery shelves . . .

Aspartame

EqualTM and NutraSweetTM are the actual marketed names of aspartame. Aspartame enhances the taste of sweeteners and is about 200 times sweeter than sucrose. A molecule of aspartame consists of two amino acids (phenylalanine and aspartic acid) linked by a molecule of methanol, the alcohol found in antifreeze. At 86 degrees F, lower than your body temperature, these components break down and have distinctive effects. The methanol is metabolized by your body to formaldehyde and then to formic acid. Both of these are potent metabolic poisons. Phenylalanine and aspartic acid both mimic brain neurotransmitters and can upset the balance of chemicals and may be linked to depression, seizures, memory problems, Parkinson's, ALS, multiple sclerosis, and the onset of adult diabetes.

BHA

Butylated hydroxyanisole is used as a preservative in baked goods, candy, chewing gum, soup bases, breakfast cereals, shortening, dry mixes for cakes, potatoes, potato flakes, and ice cream. BHA is also an antioxidant and may affect liver and kidney function. BHA has been associated with children's behavioural problems.

BHT	Butylated hydroxytoluene retards rancidity in frozen and fresh pork sausage and freeze-dried meats. The base product used in shortenings and animal fats contains BHT. It is also the base product for chewing gum. Allergic reactions and enlargement of the liver can be side effects of BHT.
Caffeine	Caffeine is a stimulant and is addictive. Consuming large amounts of caffeine over a long period of time can have toxic effects on the body and can affect blood sugar release, the liver, the central nervous system, the heart, and the respiratory system. Caffeine can cause irregular heartbeats, insomnia, irritability, and mood swings. Caffeine is an ingredient in coffee, tea, soft drinks, and chocolate.
Nitrates and Nitrites	Nitrates are natural occuring chemicals, and are used to preserve meat and to improve flavour.

Nitrates (also called nitrites) in large amounts are known to be toxic and can cause cancer. Years ago, manufacturers used to add sodium nitrite to baby food to make it look better. Once the public became aware of the risks of nitrites in food, the industry withdrew the nitrites in the baby foods.

The meat industry says that nitrites are needed to inhibit the growth of bacteria that cause botulism. It is important to know that nitrites do not destroy bacteria spores but only retard their germination. Proper refrigeration and adhering to throw-away dates would work just as well. Studies have shown that manufacturers could add vitamin C or E to processed meats as an added protection. Perhaps with increased public awareness of the dangers of additives such as nitrites, the government would seek out alternative methods.

Sorbate	Sorbate is a fungus preventative and preservative found in chocolate syrups, deli salads, cheesecake, pie fillings, preserves, baked goods, and artificially sweetened jellies. Researchers have found that this chemical interrupts enzyme functions, and since the human body has many enzyme systems, any interference could cause problems.

Sulfites are used to reduce and prevent discolouration of vegetables and fruits such as dried fruits and dehydrated potatoes. They are a preservative and bleaching agent and they are found in sliced fruit, beer, and wine. They are also found in salad dressings, gravies, corn syrup, wine vinegar, and sauces. Reactions to sulfites may include hives, dizziness, difficulty in breathing, and, in rare instances, even death.

Sugar is one of the most damaging and destructive items in our daily diets. Sugar in any form is very quickly absorbed into the blood stream and it may provide quick energy, but it is short-lived. Remember that sugar, whether it is from the cane, sugar beets, or from corn, has no nutritional value and provides empty calories. The body converts all sugars to glucose, and once converted, it is circulated through the blood stream as an energy source and stored in the liver and muscles as fat.

Sugar is addictive and acts like a drug when eaten in large amounts or consumed daily. Remember that fruit juices are very high in natural sugars and can have the same harmful effects as pure sugar. Sugar is everywhere in your diet. North Americans consume on an average 130 pounds of sugar and sweeteners per year. The average person consumes 20% of his/her calories from some form of refined sugar. This high consumption of sugar is a relatively new finding, becoming a staple in our diet in the past two centuries. In Colonial America, table sugar cost $2.40 per pound as opposed to the low cost of approximately fifty cents per pound today.

Upon ingestion of sugar, the immune system is almost immediately depressed — i.e. it becomes weaker — and this can predispose people to infections and allergies. Influenza (Flu) and other respiratory infections can often be traced to heavy sugar consumption, especially after holidays, when a lot of sweets are consumed. The minerals needed to digest sugar are chromium, manganese, cobalt, copper, zinc, and magnesium. These have been stripped away in the sugar refining process, and the body has to deplete its own mineral reserves to process the refined sugar.

Sugar also creates an imbalance of the calcium/phosphorus ratio, causing blood levels of calcium to increase and phosphorus to decrease (this can mean that blood levels of calcium will remain in the normal range while the person may be developing osteoporosis). The sugar causes an increase in calcium excretion from the body. Even just two teaspoons of sugar can change the mineral ratios in our body.

Names of forms of sugar:

Sucrose	Brown Sugar
Dextrose	Lactose
Sorbitol	Molasses
Corn syrup	Invert Sugar
Fructose	Xylitol
Maltose	Glucose
Honey	

Some commercially available foods containing sugar:

Ketchup
(1 tbsp ketchup contains 1 tsp of sugar)

Soft Drinks
(some contain up to 12 tsp of sugar per 8 ounces)

Jelly Beans and Marshmallows
(these are 100% sugar)

Gravies

Mayonnaise

Sauces

Processed Meats

Cereals

Relish

TV Dinner

Peanut Butter

Mustard

Breads

Some Drugs

Substitutes for
Common Foods

Now that you know you have food allergies and/or intolerances, you need to know what you can eat. Here is a list of substitutes for common foods and how much is needed in a recipe to substitute. Also, here are suggestions for some new foods such as grains and lentils and how to cook them. For me, many of these foods were new, and I was at a loss to know where to buy them, what to cook with them, and how to cook them.

Food alternatives

Dairy products

1 cup (250 ml)	Cow's Milk =	
1 cup (250 ml)	Goat's Milk	
1 cup (250 ml)	Soy Milk	
1 cup (250 ml)	Rice Milk	
1 cup (250 ml)	Nut Milk	
1 cup (250 ml)	Hemp Milk	
1/4 cup (50 ml)	Tofu blended with 3/4 cup (175 ml) water	
1/3 cup (75 ml)	Shredded Coconut blended with 1 cup (250 ml) water	
1/4 cup (50 ml)	Nuts or Seeds blended with 1 cup (250 ml) water	
1 cup Buttermilk	= 1 cup (250 ml) Soy Milk with 2 tsp (10 ml) lemon juice.	

Alternatives

Soy Milk

Rice Milk

Nut Milk

Hemp Milk

Coconut Milk

Goat's Milk

(Some people who cannot tolerate cow's milk can tolerate goat's milk.)

Eggs

1	Egg =
1 Tbsp (15 ml)	ground flaxseed with 3-4 Tbsp (45-60 ml) water; put in blender or whisk (use as a binder)
1 Tbsp (15 ml)	ground chia seed with 3-4 Tbsp (45-60 ml) water; put in blender or whisk (use as a binder)
1 Tbsp (15 ml)	unground flaxseed in 3/4 cup (175 ml) water, put in pot, bring to boil for 5 minutes, let simmer and cool down a bit, then add to muffins as a binder
1/4 cup (50 ml)	tofu for each egg replacer (use as a binder)
1 Tbsp (15 ml)	soften Gelatin in 3 Tbsp (45 ml) boiling water, stir until dissolved, put in freezer; take out when thickened and beat until frothy (use as a binder)
1 tsp (5 ml)	baking powder for each egg (use for leavening)
1 Tbsp (15 ml)	psyllium husk with 3 Tbsp (45 ml) water and let sit briefly
1/4 tsp (1 ml)	Guar Gum
1 egg white=	1/4 tsp (1 ml) Agar Agar in 2 Tbsp (30 ml) water, whip, chill, and whip

Alternatives

Tofu

Commercial Egg Replacer

Gelatin

Flaxseed

Chia Seed

Psyllium Husk

Agar Flakes

Arrowroot

Mashed Banana

Duck eggs or quail eggs are sometimes tolerated by those allergic to chicken eggs.

Butter

Instead of spreading butter, try tahini, tofu, mashed avocado, nut butters, or lentil spreads. Try olive oil, safflower, sunflower, sesame, avocado, or coconut oil to replace butter in recipes.

Flours

1 cup (250 ml)	White or Wheat Flour =
1 cup (250 ml)	**Spelt Flour**
1 cup (250 ml)	**Millet Flour**
7/8 cup (220 ml)	**Buckwheat Flour (1 cup (250 ml) minus 2 Tbsp (30 ml))**
7/8 cup (220 ml)	**Rice Flour**
3/4 cup (175 ml)	**Brown Rice Flour**
1 cup (250 ml)	**Soybean Flour**
1 cup (250 ml)	**Rye Flour**
3/4 cup (175 ml)	**Barley Flour**
3/4 cup (175 ml)	**Chickpea Flour or other bean flour**
1 cup (250 ml)	**Oat Flour**
1 cup (250 ml)	**Tapioca Flour**
7/8 cup (220 ml)	**Kamut, Quinoa, or Amaranth Flour**
1 cup (250 ml)	**Cassava Flour**

Thickeners

1 Tbsp (15 ml)	Wheat Flour =
1 1/2 Tbsp (22 ml)	**Arrowroot**
1/2 Tbsp (7 ml)	**Cornstarch**
1 Tbsp (15 ml)	**Spelt Flour**
1 Tbsp (15 ml)	**Tapioca Flour**
1 Tbsp (15 ml)	**Potato Flour or Potato Starch**

Alternatives to wheat

Amaranth

Barley

Buckwheat

Brown Rice

Cassava

Chickpea

Kamut

Millet

Oat

Quinoa

Rye

Soy

Spelt

Tapioca

Teff

Sugar

1 cup (250 ml)	Sugar =
1/2 cup (125 ml)	Agave Nectar
1/2 cup (125 ml)	Honey
1/2 cup (125 ml)	Maple Syrup
1/2 cup (125 ml)	Molasses
1/2 cup (125 ml)	Rice Syrup
3/4 cup (175 ml)	Barley Malt
1/2 cup (125 ml)	Fruit Purée
1 tsp (5 ml)	ground Stevia
1/2 cup (125ml)	date sugar
1/2 cup (125ml)	coconut sugar

Alternatives

Stevia

Maple Syrup

Honey

Molasses

Rice Syrup

Fruit Juice

Barley Malt

Fruit

Note

If you feel the need to use a sweetener, try using pure maple syrup, rice syrup, barley malt, molasses, honey, or stevia. All can be found in your local health food store.

Stevia is a natural alternative to sugar. It is from a plant that grows in Paraguay and it is 300 times sweeter than sugar. For years, Paraguayans have used the leaves of the stevia plant to make sweet teas and to sweeten their foods.

Stevia has antifungal properties, is beneficial in fat absorption, and does not affect blood-sugar levels or promote tooth decay. Stevia plants are available in Canada and can be grown here in the summer months. Check with your local organic farmers' market. If you are using stevia leaves to sweeten your tea, one or two leaves should be ample. If you are using ground stevia for baking, 1 1/2 - 2 teaspoons (7-10 ml) are equivalent to 1 cup (250 ml) of sugar. Each plant can differ in sweetness, so use your judgment and taste the powder first.

Coconut sugar does not put stress on your blood sugar the same way white sugar does.

Vinegar

Lemon or lime juice, cranberry juice, or dilute 1 teaspoon (5 ml) of Vitamin C crystals in 1/4 cup (50 ml) water. Some people use apple cider vinegar, which they can tolerate as it is the corn in the white vinegar that bothers some.

Pie bases

Ground nuts or seeds, mashed vegetables, mashed sweet potato or regular potato.

Tops of pies

Sweet potato, white potato, grated fruit or vegetables.

Raising agents

Try to avoid commercial baking powder, as it contains cornstarch, gluten, and aluminum. Buy aluminum-free baking powder or make your own baking powder. Mix together 1 teaspoon (5 ml) bicarbonate of soda and 2 teaspoons (10 ml) cream of tartar. Use 1 teaspoon (5 ml) of this mixture for each cup of flour called for in the recipe. Or try 1/4 teaspoon (1 ml) baking soda and 1/2 teaspoon (2 ml) lemon or lime juice or powdered Vitamin C crystals.

Unbuffered Vitamin C crystals are used in conjunction with baking soda to help leaven. They can also be used in salads instead of vinegar or lemon juice.

Gelatin

Agar Flakes. Agar is derived from seaweed and can be used instead of gelatin. It is available in flakes or powder and usually it takes less of the powder than of the flakes to produce jelling.

Chocolate

Carob powder or carob chips. Carob comes from the legume family and is a good substitute for chocolate.

White bread

100% rye bread or sourdough bread, spelt, barley, kamut, or rice bread.

Vegetable oil

Cold-pressed oils: sunflower oil, safflower oil, canola oil, flax oil, virgin olive oil. Try for organic oils if you can.

White rice

Brown rice, basmati rice, wild rice.

Soda crackers

Rye or rice crackers, rice cakes. For breadings and coatings you can also grind any nuts or seeds.

Wheat pasta

Corn pasta, kamut pasta, quinoa pasta, spelt pasta, rice pasta.

White potato

Sweet potato, rice, yams, noodles, carrots, corn, squash, pumpkin, rutabaga, turnips, parsnips, radishes, onions, beans, shallots, kohlrabi.

Definitions

Nightshades

The nightshade family includes white potato, tobacco, and peppers of all kinds, including pimiento, paprika, cayenne, and chili. White and black pepper are not part of the nightshade family.

Gluten

A protein found in grains such as wheat, oats, spelt, rye, triticale, and couscous. When mixed with a liquid, it produces elasticity in dough and helps it to rise. If you have been told to stay away from gluten, here are some alternate suggestions:

Flours: Corn, rice, buckwheat, millet, tapioca, teff, quinoa, soy, potato, arrowroot, amaranth, or chickpea.

Pastas: Rice, corn, quinoa, or buckwheat.

Cereals: Try puffed rice, puffed corn, puffed amaranth, or quinoa. You can also have peas, beans, lentils, nuts, and seeds.

Different types of grains

Amaranth* Meaning "immortal" in Greek, amaranth contains the highest protein of any grain and is rich in lysine, an essential amino acid that many grains lack. It contains a more complete protein than either milk or soybeans and is a good source of fibre. Amaranth is ideal for vegetarians, because it's high in both proteins and minerals but low in fats and cholesterol. Amaranth is a good alternative grain for those allergic to wheat, as the flour can be substituted in almost any recipe and is excellent in baked goods. Amaranth seeds can be popped like popcorn and can be used in energy bars. When amaranth seeds are boiled in water and then chilled, they develop a gelatinous texture, so they can be used to prepare jams and fruit spreads without the use of pectin and/or sweetener. Amaranth is gluten-free.

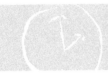 For a hot breakfast cereal, cook 1 cup (250 ml) whole amaranth seed in 2 cups (500 ml) of water, simmer slowly, and add more water as needed. Sweeten with honey and add some soy milk or rice milk.

Barley Barley is a partially refined food, as the outer layers are removed because they are very tough. Pearl barley has been refined until it is small and white, so pot barley is preferred as it contains more nutrients. Barley has a delightful flavour, is chewy and is nice added to soups. It is a good source of protein, potassium, and other minerals. Barley flour can be substituted in recipes that call for wheat flour and is great in pie crusts.

Barley was brought to North America from Europe, where it was grown to be used in the making of beer. People swear by it for bladder infections. Simmer a half cup barley in six cups of water for three hours, strain and use the barley for soup. Add lemon juice and honey to the liquid and drink it.

 To cook whole barley, use 1 cup (250 ml) barley to 3 cups (750 ml) water and cook for 75 minutes.

Buckwheat*

Buckwheat contains almost as much protein as eggs but no cholesterol and is high in potassium and B vitamins and is gluten-free. Buckwheat is not related to the wheat family and can usually be tolerated by people who are allergic to wheat. Buckwheat is actually a seed, rich in a flavonoid glycoside known as rutin. Rutin aids in the treatment of high blood pressure and hardening of the arteries. It is good for using in cake recipes and for pancakes or crepes.

 To cook buckwheat use 1 cup (250 ml) buckwheat to 2 cups (500 ml) water and cook for 15 minutes.

Bulgur

Bulgur is simply whole wheat grains that have been soaked and cooked until cracked, hence it is also known as cracked wheat.

To cook, use 1 cup (250 ml) bulgur wheat to 2 cups (500 ml) water and cook for 20 minutes.

Kamut

Kamut has a rich, buttery flavour and has true "energy properties."

The story says that kamut was taken from an Egyptian tomb and hence it has been called "King Tut's wheat." It is a relative of durum wheat and is a member of the grass family, so it can be tolerated by people who have a wheat allergy. Kamut is higher in minerals and proteins than wheat and is high in magnesium and zinc. It has no fat or cholesterol but does contain gluten. Kamut is great as a pasta and to me tastes very much like regular wheat pasta. Kamut flakes also work well in granola if you are trying to avoid oats.

Millet*

Millet is full of nutrients — proteins, vitamins, and minerals — and is gluten-free. It has a lovely nutty flavour and is an alkaline grain easy to digest and is non-mucus-forming, so it is great for babies and the elderly. Millet is a grain that is least likely to affect people with sensitivities. Cook it the same way you do rice. The best millet is a golden colour. Millet flour can be used for baked goods but can sometimes come out crumbly.

 To bring out its nutty flavour, dry roast the grain in a cast iron pan for 5 minutes before cooking. Use 2 cups (500 ml) water for each cup (250 ml) of millet. Cook approximately 30 minutes.

Oats

Oats are full of nutrients. They are high in silica, good for the complexion and shiny hair. Oat groats are the whole, hulled grain, and rolled oats are oat groats rolled flat so that they cook faster. Instant oatmeal has been precooked, so not a great idea.

 Use 1 cup (250 ml) rolled oats to 3 cups (750 ml) water and simmer for 30 minutes. Use 1 cup (250 ml) whole oats to 5 cups (1.25 l) water and cook for several hours.

Quinoa*

Pronounced "keenwa," it is known as the mother grain. It is grown in Canada organically and is a good source of nutrition. It is high in protein and has natural sugars, essential fatty acids, B vitamins, and trace minerals. Quinoa contains all eight of the essential amino acids, making it a high-quality protein. It is very versatile and can be used in many recipes as well as being gluten-free. Rinse well before cooking.

 Use 1 cup (250 ml) quinoa to 2 cups (500 ml) water. Bring to a boil and then reduce to simmer for 15 minutes.

Rice*

Rice is low in fat and provides protein and most of the B vitamins. Brown rice is the whole grain with the husk removed and the rest of the kernel intact, which includes the bran and the germ, and is very easily digested. Short-grain rice has a softer, stickier texture when cooked and is good to use in puddings or sauces. Long-grain rice is drier. Basmati rice is chewier and gives a wonderful aroma when cooking. Wild rice is not a rice, but seeds from grass. It is very nutritious and has more protein than oats or brown rice and is high in minerals. When rice is served with legumes, you have a healthy meal, high in protein, low in fat and cholesterol, and high in vitamins and minerals.

 When cooking brown rice, use 1 cup (250 ml) rice to 2 cups (500 ml) water, bring to boil and simmer for 40 minutes.

Rye

Rye has a low gluten content, so rye bread does not rise as much as other breads and it usually fills you up faster. Rye is high in protein and has a distinctive flavour. It is very versatile and can be substituted well for recipes that call for wheat. Cracked rye is great as a breakfast cereal.

To cook rye, use 1 cup (250 ml) rye to 3 cups (750 ml) water and cook for 60 minutes.

Spelt

Spelt is a grain that was grown in Europe over 9,000 years ago. Some people with wheat allergies can tolerate spelt. It contains more protein, fat, and fibre than wheat and is rich in Vitamins A and B, potassium, and trace minerals. Some research shows that it helps blood to clot and stimulates the immune system. Spelt flour is excellent in baked goods such as breads and muffins. Spelt flour is drier than wheat flour, so you may need to adjust your recipe with a bit more liquid or oil.

To cook spelt grain, use 1 cup (250 ml) spelt to 1 1/2 cups (375 ml) water and cook for 30 minutes.

Teff*

An ancient grain of Ethiopia, teff comes in both ivory and dark teff. It has a lovely taste and is great in cookies, muffins, and pancakes, and is gluten-free. Teff is a good source of iron, calcium, and B vitamins. Look for teff grain and flour in the bulk sections of your local health food store. Like other grains, it should be stored in a cool, dry place or in the refrigerator or freezer.

To cook teff grain, use 1 cup (250 ml) teff to 3 cups (750 ml) water and cook for 20 minutes.

Notes

* Grains that are gluten-free.

Wheat   Wheat is the universal grain. It has a high gluten content, therefore is good for making breads. When buying wheat flour, make sure it says stone ground, otherwise it will have been processed differently with most of the nutritious content gone and can go rancid quickly. Flours should be used quickly once ground to avoid going rancid or should be kept in the freezer. Soft wheat is a golden colour, and hard wheat is brown or red in colour.

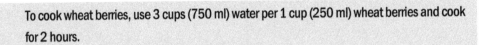

To cook wheat berries, use 3 cups (750 ml) water per 1 cup (250 ml) wheat berries and cook for 2 hours.

A few hints about beans

You have all heard the tune "Beans, beans, the magical fruit, the more you eat 'em, the more you toot." Here are a few hints when cooking beans to avoid the toots.

- Rinse beans thoroughly. Pick over and discard any discoloured beans or stones. Most beans should be soaked overnight and then rinsed a couple of times before cooking. Lentils do not need to be pre-soaked.

- Combine beans with prescribed amount of water and bring water to a boil, skim off foam, reduce heat, and cover.

- If you can squish 'em with your fingers, the beans are done.

- If you wish to add sea salt, do so at the end of the cooking period, otherwise it will cause the legumes to toughen. Rinse your beans well after cooking. Remember that dried beans double in volume as they cook.

- To help get rid of flatulence, you can cook legumes with a piece of washed kombu (seaweed).

- You can also add summer savory, cumin, caraway seeds, or fennel when cooking beans, as these herbs help to reduce bean flatulence as well.

Different types of legumes

Legumes are an excellent source of fibre. By introducing legumes and grains into your diet, you will have more options and variety, especially if you need to avoid beef, chicken, or pork, or simply wish a more vegetarian type diet.

Legume (1 cup (250 ml) dry measure)	Water	Cooking Time	Yield
Aduki Beans	4 cups (1 l)	1 hour	2 cups (500 ml)
Black Beans	4 cups (1 l)	1 1/2 hours	2 cups (500 ml)
Chickpeas (Garbanzos)	4 cups (1 l)	3 hours	2 cups (500 ml)
Great Northern Beans	3 1/2 cups (875 ml)	2 hours	2 cups (500 ml)
Kidney Beans	3 cups (750 ml)	1 1/2 hours	2 cups (500 ml)
Lima Beans	2 cups (500 ml)	1 1/2 hours	1 1/4 cups (300 ml)
Mung Beans	3 cups (750 ml)	1 hour	3 cups (750 ml)
Pinto and Navy Beans	3 cups (750 ml)	2 hours	2 cups (500 ml)
Soybeans	4 cups (1 l)	3 hours	2 cups (500 ml)
Split Peas	3 cups (750 ml)	45 minutes	2 1/4 cups (550 ml)
Lentils	3 cups (750 ml)	30 minutes	2 1/4 cups (550 ml)

Basic Food

Combining

General food combining

Food combining is not new, but with today's fast-paced society it can sometimes be hard to implement. The basic idea behind food combining is that better digestion and absorption of foods are obtained by combining certain foods in a meal and not others. Each food has its own rate of digestion and absorption. Foods are broken down into unique components consisting of proteins, carbohydrates, and fats. For optimum digestion, it would be best to eat every food alone, but for variety we mix our foods, and so it is important to know which foods are best mixed with others.

The main principle of food combining is that starch foods and protein foods are not eaten at the same meal. So no meat and potatoes, rice and fish, bread and cheese.

Improper food combining places an enormous burden on the digestive system and this can tire you out even more than you already are if you have food sensitivities.

Foods break down in different parts of the intestines, so it is important to try to combine foods that will break down together. For example, if you eat some sunflower seeds, which break down in the stomach, and then you eat an orange immediately, the following will happen: the orange will get held up in the stomach with the seeds, it will start to ferment, and gas will result. The orange will therefore start to "rot" before it can be absorbed by your digestive tract.

Many people will find that with proper food combining they will have less gas, heartburn, and bloating after meals. You may also find that you will have better bowel movements, which may help you to shed some excess pounds if you are overweight.

Some basic rules for food combining are to eat fruits alone. Do not eat proteins with starches; green vegetables go well with proteins or starches.

Please see the attached chart for food combining.

Remember, your body is your best judge. Some people's systems can handle more than others. Each person is unique and has a different constitution. Do what is best for you and what makes you feel the best.

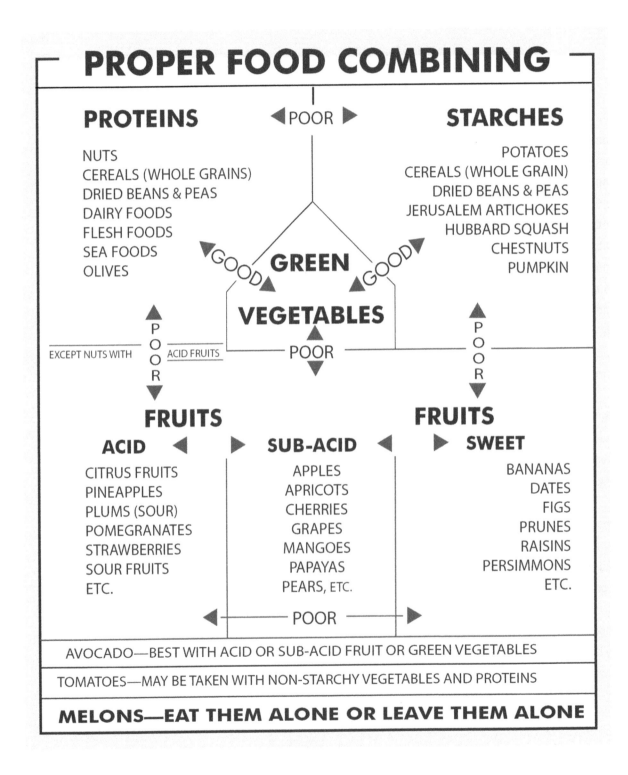

PROPER FOOD COMBINING

PROTEINS ◀ POOR ▶ STARCHES

PROTEINS

NUTS
CEREALS (WHOLE GRAINS)
DRIED BEANS & PEAS
DAIRY FOODS
FLESH FOODS
SEA FOODS
OLIVES

STARCHES

POTATOES
CEREALS (WHOLE GRAIN)
DRIED BEANS & PEAS
JERUSALEM ARTICHOKES
HUBBARD SQUASH
CHESTNUTS
PUMPKIN

◀ GOOD ▶ GREEN ◀ GOOD ▶

VEGETABLES

POOR

POOR — EXCEPT NUTS WITH — ACID FRUITS

POOR

FRUITS   **FRUITS**

ACID ◀   ▶ **SUB-ACID** ◀   ▶ **SWEET**

ACID

CITRUS FRUITS
PINEAPPLES
PLUMS (SOUR)
POMEGRANATES
STRAWBERRIES
SOUR FRUITS
ETC.

SUB-ACID

APPLES
APRICOTS
CHERRIES
GRAPES
MANGOES
PAPAYAS
PEARS, ETC.

SWEET

BANANAS
DATES
FIGS
PRUNES
RAISINS
PERSIMMONS
ETC.

◀ POOR ▶

AVOCADO—BEST WITH ACID OR SUB-ACID FRUIT OR GREEN VEGETABLES

TOMATOES—MAY BE TAKEN WITH NON-STARCHY VEGETABLES AND PROTEINS

MELONS—EAT THEM ALONE OR LEAVE THEM ALONE

Helpful Hints
to the Cook

Cooking times are approximate, as variations in oven temperatures do occur. Always preheat your oven to the specified temperature before placing dish in the oven.

Please note that not all recipes have been tried with all substitutes and so if the recipe calls for oat flour pay attention to the note section in "substituting" if you are to use a different flour. Some flours can make recipes drier than others, as does using different egg substitutes. Under each recipe it states whether this recipe is free of dairy, wheat, yeast, corn, sugar, eggs, soy, nuts, nightshades, and gluten. When I refer to sugar, I mean refined white sugar. The recipe still may contain sugar, but it will be in the form of fruit, maple syrup, honey, brown rice syrup, or alternatives like stevia.

When I refer to wheat free in a recipe I mean whole wheat. Spelt and Kamut are ancient forms of wheat, but many people who cannot tolerate white flour or whole wheat flour can tolerate spelt and kamut. If you need to avoid all wheat or gluten, you need to avoid spelt and kamut as well.

- Try to purchase organic produce whenever possible. The use of pesticides is rampant in North America and it is best to avoid store-bought produce unless they offer organic.

- Buy from your local organic grower or natural food store.

- Try to use filtered water if you can. It is best to avoid the chlorine in the water and other nasties that are usually present in your local water.

- Try to purchase freshly ground flours and keep them in the refrigerator or freezer.

- All nuts, grains, and seeds should be kept refrigerated so they don't go rancid.

- Before cooking beans, remember to soak them and discard the water; this will help avoid flatulence — or the toots, as we call them in our family! You can also add a piece of washed kombu (seaweed) while soaking and cooking your legumes, as it, too, helps in ridding the legumes of gaseous enzymes.

- If you are tired when you are making cookies, wrap the cookie dough in wax paper, on the unwaxed side, and put in the fridge until the next day when you have more energy to finish baking.

- Parchment paper is great to put on cookie sheets so the baking does not burn and it helps the baking to retain its moisture while cooking. It is safe and non-toxic, too.

- Use cooked chickpeas in vegetarian spaghetti sauce to thicken it and to add protein instead of using meat. You might also try TVP (textured vegetable protein).

- Use cooked beets in your spaghetti sauce to sweeten it instead of using sugar. Purée the beets before adding them to the sauce.

- You can also use beet water as a natural food colouring for cakes, icings, and puddings.

- Use a crockpot. You can start it at night, and in the morning you have cooked grains ready to eat. Start dinner in the morning — bean soups or chilis or even a pot roast or chicken.

- Try using fresh herbs as they add much more flavor than dried herbs

- Use a coffee grinder to grind seeds, nuts, or spices.

- If you buy fresh ginger, wrap it and keep it in the freezer. It will last longer than in the fridge. I find that fresh ginger after a week in the fridge will start to turn mouldy. Simply remove from freezer, grate, and use.

- If you find you are losing weight because there are many foods you can no longer eat, try eating more nuts and seeds. Oils contain twice as many calories as starches and proteins. Avocados have healthy fat, and flaxseed oil is good to sprinkle on salads and cooked vegetables. Have snacks between meals, like trail mixes or rice crackers with yummy avocado spread or bean pâte on them.

- Try to use organic cold-pressed oils.

- Stuck for breakfast ideas because you can no longer eat dairy, eggs, wheat, or yeast? Don't limit yourself. Be nontraditional and have fish or rice for breakfast. Eat whatever you can and don't feel pressured because you can no longer eat bacon, eggs, and toast.

- Edible flowers are great on a salad; grow them in your garden. Just make sure no one uses pesticides in your neighbourhood, as the wind carries the pesticides quite a distance when they are sprayed.

- Try to use only sea salt, as table salt is refined and sometimes has added sugar in it.

- Try expeller-pressed, unrefined safflower or sunflower oil in dessert baking if you have to omit butter, or instead of using margarine.

- Try to purchase natural vanilla extract. There is vanilla extract (from boiling down the vanilla bean) and vanilla essence (from soaking the bean in alcohol and adding caramel colouring).

- Try Tofutti ice cream or Tofutti Cuties; they are dairy-free ice creams.

- Rice Dream ice cream is made from rice and is a dairy-free ice cream.

Now Let's get on to the recipes!

Please note: According to the Canadian Food and Drug Inspection Agency, a food containing spelt or kamut is not considered to be wheat-free. This may vary for each country. Please always read labels or check with your health care provider.

Breakfast

and Juices

48   Muesli

49   Maple Granola

50   Rice Porridge with Ginger and Blueberries

51   Banana Oatmeal

52   Hot Cereal

53   Fig Butter

54   Spelt Pancakes

55   Blueberry Buckwheat Pancakes

56   Quinoa Pancakes

57   Yummy Teff Pancakes

58   Millet Applejacks

59   Morning Quinoa

60   Scrambled Tofu

61   Applesauce Breakfast Cake

62   Squash Cranberry Muffins

63   Juice for Candida

63   Juice for increasing your Potassium

63   Cleansing Juice

63   Calcium-rich Juice

63   Some Other Juicing Ideas

Muesli

Free of dairy products, wheat, yeast, corn, sugar, eggs, nightshades and gluten. Can be soy free if you use rice milk.

Ingredients

1/4 cup	gluten-free rolled oats (50ml)
1/4 cup	gluten-free oat bran (50ml)
2 Tbsp	raisins (30 ml)
1 Tbsp	chopped walnuts (15 ml)
1 tsp	organic lemon zest, grated (5 ml)
1	organic apple, grated
	Soy milk, rice milk, or nut milk
	Seasonal fruit (blueberries, strawberries, peaches, raspberries)

- In your blender or food processor, blend oats, oat bran, raisins, walnuts, and grated lemon.

- Transfer to a bowl, add choice of milk and fruit, mix, and enjoy.

Yields 1 serving.

NOTE

You can substitute wheat germ or corn germ instead of oat bran. You can also substitute dates for raisins and add grated coconut instead of walnuts or add a banana as your fruit.

Maple Granola

Free of dairy products, wheat, yeast, corn, sugar, eggs, soy, nightshades and gluten. For a nut-free granola, leave out the almonds.

- Mix all ingredients together in a bowl except dried fruit. You can purchase sliced almonds or simply buy whole almonds and slice them in your food processor.

- Spread onto a cookie sheet and bake at 350F for 20 minutes or until golden.

- Stir occasionally. When brown, remove from oven and stir in raisins or dried fruit and mix well.

- Let cool and store granola in glass jar in the refrigerator.

Yields 4 cups (1 L).

Ingredients

2/3 cup	gluten-free rolled oats (150ml)
2/3 cup	gluten-free oat bran (150ml)
3/4 cup	grated coconut (175 ml)
1/2 cup	sunflower seeds (125 ml)
1/4 cup	sesame seeds (50 ml)
1 cup	sliced almonds (250 ml)
1/2 cup	safflower or coconut oil (125 ml)
1/4 cup	maple syrup (50 ml)
1 1/2 cups	raisins or dried fruit (375 ml)
1 Tbsp	flaxseed or chia seed (15 ml)

Rice Porridge with Ginger and Blueberries

Free of dairy products, wheat, yeast, corn, sugar, eggs, soy, nightshades, and gluten. For a nut-free porridge, leave out the nuts.

Ingredients

2 cups	cooked short-grain organic brown rice (500 ml)
	Handful of pecans or walnuts
	Handful of fresh or frozen blueberries
	Maple syrup to taste
1/2 tsp	fresh ginger, grated (2 ml)
	Water

- Place nuts in a dry cast iron pan and over medium heat roast for a few minutes. Shake the pan frequently so they don't burn. Remove nuts and put aside. If you don't have time to roast nuts, just leave them as they are.

- Combine cooked rice and water in a saucepan over medium heat and simmer for 5-10 minutes, stirring frequently until thick porridge consistency. Use enough water to make it goopy.

- Wash blueberries and place them in a saucepan over medium heat with maple syrup and ginger for a few minutes to heat through.

- In a bowl, place warm rice, berries, and nuts on top, and enjoy. Serve hot.

  This is one of my favourites for breakfast. I try to plan ahead and the night before if I cook brown rice for dinner, I make sure I cook a little extra for breakfast the next day.

Yields 2 cups (500 ml).

NOTE
You can substitute cinnamon for ginger.

Banana Oatmeal

Free of dairy products, wheat, yeast, corn, sugar, eggs, soy, nuts, nightshades and gluten.

- Bring apple cider and water to a boil. Stir in remaining ingredients except blueberries.

- Cook on medium heat for 15-20 minutes or until done.

- Top with blueberries.

- Serve hot.

Yields 1 large serving.

Ingredients

1/3 cup	gluten-free rolled oats (75ml)
1 Tbsp	ground flax seeds (15 ml)
1/2 cup	cooked short-grain organic brown rice (125 ml)
3/4 cups	apple cider or apple juice (175 ml)
1/4 cup	water (50 ml)
1/2	mashed banana
	Handful of blueberries (optional)

Hot Cereal

Ingredients

1/2 cup	ground grains, such as amaranth, oat groats, buckwheat groats, rye, millet, or teff (125 ml)
1 1/2 cups	water, apple cider, or fruit juice (375 ml)
	Handful of organic Thompson raisins
	Chopped almonds, walnuts, or pecans
1 Tbsp	sesame or sunflower seeds (15 ml)

Free of dairy products, wheat, yeast, corn, sugar, eggs, soy, and nightshades, and can be gluten free if you use millet, teff, or buckwheat. Again, nuts can be optional.

- Bring water or juice to a boil with the raisins, seeds, and nuts, then add in the grains and stir constantly.

- Simmer for 30 minutes or until desired texture and serve.

- Top with cinnamon and flaxseed oil or applesauce.

Yields 2 servings.

Fig Butter

Free of dairy products, wheat, yeast, corn, sugar, eggs, soy, nuts, nightshades, and gluten.

Ingredients

1 1/2 cups	dried figs, chopped (375 ml)
1 cup	apple juice (250 ml)
	Pinch cinnamon
	Juice and grated zest of 1 lemon

- In a saucepan combine figs, apple juice, cinnamon, lemon zest, and juice.

- Cover and simmer until figs are soft, about 45 minutes.

- Purée in food processor. Delicious as a spread for toast.

- Keep in a glass jar in the fridge.

Yields 1 1/2 cups (375 ml).

DID YOU KNOW?
That figs are rich in complex carbohydrates, a good source of dietary fibre, and rich in essential minerals such as potassium, iron, and calcium. Half a cup of figs will give you as much calcium as half a cup of milk, and because they have no fat, cholesterol, or sodium, they make a great snack.

Spelt Pancakes

Free of dairy products, wheat, yeast, corn, sugar, eggs, nuts, and nightshades. This can be soy free if you use rice milk instead.

Ingredients

1 cup	spelt flour (250 ml)
1 Tbsp	honey (optional) (15 ml)
2 tsp	baking powder (10ml)
	Pinch salt
1 cup	soy milk or rice milk (250 ml)
2 Tbsp	safflower or coconut oil (30 ml)

- Combine flour, baking powder, and salt in bowl and mix well.

- Mix in soy milk, oil, and honey, and whisk until smooth.

- Pour batter onto a hot, oiled frying pan to form small-sized pancakes.

- When bubbles appear, flip pancake and cook for another 2 minutes. Serve with fruit or maple syrup.

Yields 10 small pancakes.

NOTE

You can also use half brown rice flour, half spelt flour in this recipe. Try adding some blueberries or a pinch of cinnamon to the batter.

DID YOU KNOW?

That spelt contains special carbohydrates (mucopolysaccharides), which stimulate the body's immune system; and is an excellent source of protein.

Blueberry Buckwheat Pancakes

Free of dairy products, wheat, yeast, corn, sugar, eggs, soy, nuts, nightshades, and gluten.

- Mix all ingredients together in a bowl. Your batter should run but not be runny.

- Pour out pancakes onto a hot, oiled skillet and cook on medium heat until bubbles appear.

- Flip and cook until golden.

- Serve with maple syrup.

Yields 12-14 medium pancakes.

NOTE
I like to use safflower oil in my pancakes, as it is a light cooking oil and is not as heavy as olive oil.

Ingredients

1 1/2 cups	buckwheat flour (375 ml)
1/2 cup	arrowroot flour (125 ml)
1 1/2 tsp	baking soda (7 ml)
3 Tbsp	safflower or coconut oil (45 ml)
1 Tbsp	(15 ml) ground flaxseed whisked in 3 tbsp (45 ml) water
1 3/4 cup	apple juice or water (425 ml)
1 tsp	cinnamon (5 ml)
1/2 cup	blueberries (125 ml)

Quinoa Pancakes

Free of dairy products, wheat, yeast, corn, sugar, eggs, soy, nuts, nightshades, and gluten.

Ingredients

3/4 cup	quinoa flour (175 ml)
1/4 cup	tapioca flour (50 ml)
1 tsp	baking soda (5 ml)
1/4 tsp	unbuffered Vitamin C crystals (1 ml)
1/2 tsp	cinnamon (2 ml)
1/4 tsp	nutmeg (1 ml)
1 1/2-2 Tbsp	safflower or coconut oil (22-30 ml)
1 cup	apple juice (250 ml)

- In a bowl mix dry ingredients together. Add wet ingredients into dry ingredients to make a thin batter. Cook pancakes in a hot, oiled skillet until golden.

- Top with maple syrup, apple butter, or fruit.

  Quinoa has a lovely flavour, and these pancakes will be enjoyed by all.

Yields 10 small pancakes.

MY friend remarked that these were the lightest pancakes he had ever eaten.

DID YOU KNOW?
That quinoa was an ancient sacred staple food of the Incas. It contains all eight essential amino acids, making it a complete protein, and is delicious in soups and stews.

Yummy Teff Pancakes

Free of dairy products, wheat, yeast, corn, sugar, eggs, soy, nuts, nightshades, and gluten.

- Mix dry ingredients together and then mix in wet.

- Pour pancakes onto a hot, well-oiled pan, and when you see bubbles appear, flip and cook on other side.

- Serve pancakes with maple syrup or as is. If the batter is too thick, simply add a bit more apple juice.

Yields 8-10 pancakes.

NOTE

f you let this batter sit, it will tend to get thick, so you will have to add a bit more liquid to it.

These pancakes are very tasty and have a lovely dark brown colour; you can even fool your children by telling them that they are chocolate pancakes. . . for those picky eaters.

Ingredients

1 cup	teff flour (250 ml)
1 tsp	baking powder (5 ml)
1 tsp	arrowroot (5 ml)
	Pinch sea salt
1 Tbsp	safflower or coconut oil (15 ml)
3/4 cup	apple juice (175 ml)
1/2 tsp	pure vanilla extract (2 ml)

Millet Applejacks

Free of dairy products, wheat, yeast, corn, sugar, eggs, soy, nuts, and nightshades. This recipe can be egg-free if you use flaxseed.

Ingredients

1 cup	cooked millet (250 ml)
1	apple, diced
1/4 cup	oat flakes (or use quinoa, barley, spelt, or kamut) (50 ml)
1/3 cup	oat flour (or quinoa, barley, spelt, or kamut) (75 ml)
1 1/2 tsp	cinnamon (7 ml)
1/2 tsp	nutmeg (2 ml)
1	egg or flaxseed mixture
	Add water if needed
	Oil

- Mix all ingredients together. You should be able to form into patties. The mixture should be goopy, yet still hold together.

- In a hot skillet or cast-iron pan, fry applejacks in a little oil, and brown on both sides.

- Cook through for 10 minutes on a lower heat.

- Serve topped with apple butter, maple syrup, or just plain.

Yields 4 applejacks.

DID YOU KNOW?
That millet sold as bird seed has not been dehulled. Unless you have a beak, buy only hulled millet for cooking.

Morning Quinoa

Free of dairy products, wheat, yeast, corn, sugar, eggs, soy, nightshades, and gluten.

- Mix orange juice, oil, honey, and salt in a pot at medium heat.

- Rinse quinoa well and add it to the pot.

- Bring to a boil and let simmer for 20 minutes with lid on, fluff with a fork, and add roasted nuts or seeds, or raisins.

  You could also substitute apple cider or apple juice for orange juice.

Yields 1 1/2 cups (375 ml).

DID YOU KNOW?
Quinoa takes half the time to cook as brown rice.

Ingredients

1 tsp	coconut oil (5 ml)
2 tsp	honey (10 ml)
1/2 cup	quinoa (125 ml)
1 cup	orange juice (250 ml)
	Sea salt to taste
	Handful of nuts or seeds, finely chopped and roasted

Scrambled Tofu

Free of dairy products, wheat, yeast, corn, sugar, eggs, nuts, and gluten.

Ingredients

1	package tofu, 454g, patted dry and mashed
1/8 tsp	turmeric or paprika (1/2 ml)
1 tsp	onion powder (5 ml)
1/2 tsp	sea salt (2 ml)
1 cup	finely chopped red pepper, green pepper, shallots, onions, tomatoes, or whatever you like. (250 ml)

- Crumble tofu into a lightly oiled pan and cook over medium heat for 3 minutes.

- Add remaining ingredients, stir well, and cook for 5 to 8 minutes until vegetables are cooked and tofu is heated through.

Yields 4 servings.

DID YOU KNOW?

Tofu is made from curdled soy milk, an iron-rich liquid extracted from ground, cooked soybeans. It has a bland, slightly nutty flavour but tends to take on the flavour of the food with which it's cooked.

Applesauce Breakfast Cake

Free of dairy products, wheat, yeast, corn, sugar, eggs, soy, and nightshades.

- In a large saucepan heat the margarine and applesauce together over medium heat until melted, then remove from heat.

- Add remaining ingredients, stir to moisten, then pour batter into baking pan.

- Bake in a greased 9-inch square pan for 30 minutes at 350F or until a toothpick inserted comes out clean.

Yields 1 cake.

NOTE
I use spelt flour in this recipe, but you can use brown rice, barley, oat, or kamut flour, depending on your allergies.

Ingredients

1/2 cup	coconut oil (125 ml)
2 cups	unsweetened applesauce (500 ml)
1 cup	flour of your choice (250 ml)
1 1/2 cups	oat bran flakes (375 ml)
	Honey to taste
1 tsp	baking soda (5 ml)
1 1/2 tsp	cinnamon (7 ml)
1 tsp	nutmeg (5 ml)
1/4 tsp	ground cloves (1 ml)
1 cup	organic raisins (250 ml)
1 cup	chopped nuts (250 ml) (walnuts or pecans)

Squash Cranberry Muffins

Free of dairy products, wheat, yeast, corn, sugar, eggs, soy, nuts, and nightshades.

Ingredients

2 1/4 cups	spelt flour or 2 cups brown rice flour (550 ml)
1/4 cup	maple syrup (50 ml)
1 tsp	cinnamon (5 ml)
1/4 tsp	ground cloves (1 ml)
1/4 tsp	nutmeg (1 ml)
2 tsp	baking powder (10 ml)
1 tsp	baking soda (5 ml)
	Sea salt to taste
1 cup	cooked butternut squash (250 ml)
	Flaxseed mixture (1 Tbsp [15 ml] ground flaxseed with 3 Tbsp [45 ml] water, whisked)
3/4 cup	safflower oil (175 ml)
1/2 cup	vanilla rice milk or original rice milk (125 ml)
3/4 cup	cranberries (175 ml)

- In a bowl, combine flour, spices, baking powder, baking soda, and salt.

- In a separate bowl, combine mashed squash, flaxseed, oil, maple syrup, and rice milk.

- Mix well and add wet ingredients to dry. Mix, and fold in cranberries.

- Spoon into oiled muffin tin and cook at 375F for 20 minutes.

You can use any type of squash, but I prefer butternut or buttercup, as they both have lovely sweet flavours.

Yields 12 muffins.

Fruit and Vegetable Juices

Fresh fruits and vegetables are essential in order for the body to function efficiently. Many fruits and vegetables can help in the fight against certain diseases. Juicing and raw fruit diets help to eliminate wastes and toxins that have accumulated in our bodies.

It has been proven that citrus fruits containing Vitamin C and bioflavonoids help to strengthen our immune system. Fruits and vegetables that are orange in colour have higher levels of beta carotene, an anti-cancer substance that helps maintain the central nervous system and our red blood cells.

Health professionals recommend 4 to 5 servings of fruits and vegetables daily to maintain optimal health. Juicing is a great way to fill all your fruit and vegetable needs each day, so when juicing try to buy only organic produce. I find juicing is much easier if you have a juicing machine, but many juices can be made in your blender or food processor.

Here are a few juicing ideas.

Juice for Candida

1/4 inch slice fresh ginger
5 carrots, sliced
1 organic apple, sliced
Place all ingredients in your juicer and enjoy.

Juice for increasing your Potassium

Handful parsley
Handful spinach
4 carrots
2 stalks celery
For an immune builder add 1 garlic clove to recipe.
Place all ingredients in your juicer and enjoy.

Cleansing juice

1 clove garlic
1 organic beet
Organic beet greens
1 organic apple
2 organic cucumbers
Place all ingredients in your juicer and enjoy.

Calcium-rich juice

3 kale leaves
Handful fresh parsley
4 carrots
1/2 apple, seeded
Place all ingredients in your juicer and enjoy.

Some other juicing ideas:

Kale, Spinach, and Turnip Greens — a great source of Vitamin B6.
Red Swiss Chard, Turnip, Garlic, and Radish — good sources of selenium.
Parsley, Beet Greens, Dandelion Greens, Broccoli — good sources of iron.
Melon Juice: Watermelon, Cantaloupe, Orange, and Carrots.
Raspberry Juice: Raspberries, Banana, Mint.
Blueberry, Pear, and Lemon.
Grape, Apple, and Lemon.
Strawberry, Apple, and Lemon.
Strawberry and Pear.

Main Dishes
and Lunches

66   Walnut Burgers

67   Hemp Burgers

68   Bean and Rice Burgers

69   Fillings for Spelt Wraps

70   Rice Roll Ups

71   Almond Gravy

72   Salmon Croquettes

73   Ratatouille

74   Vegetarian Shepherd's Pie

76   Beef Shepherd's Pie

77   Lentil Shepherd's Pie

78   Baked Beans

80   Easy Beef or Lamb Stew

82   Stuffed Lamb

83   Pineapple Meatballs

84   Caribou Meatloaf

85   Chutney

86   Beef Stir Fry Wrapped in Lettuce Leaves

88   Stuffed Grape Leaves

89   Tuna and Pasta

90   Sweet and Sour Chicken

91   Simple Chicken Dinner

92   Garlic Shrimp with Lime

93   Barbequed Red Snapper

94   BBQ Fish Fillets

95   Fish Fingers

96   Vegetarian Tourtière

Walnut Burgers

Free of dairy products, wheat, yeast, corn, sugar, eggs, soy, and nightshades. If you use yeast-free bread, this is a yeast-free recipe.

Ingredients

1 cup	wheat-free bread crumbs (dry out toast in oven or toaster to make bread crumbs) (250 ml)
1	large onion, finely chopped and sautéed
1 tsp	sage (5 ml)
2	small cloves of garlic, minced
1/2 tsp	sea salt (2 ml)
1 cup	cooked short grain brown rice (250 ml)
1 cup	finely chopped walnuts (be sure walnuts are not bitter; if they are, they have gone rancid) (250 ml)
	Olive oil
	Water

- To cook brown rice, use 1 part rice to 2 parts water. Bring rice to a boil, cover, and simmer for 35 minutes. Once done, set rice aside to cool.

- In a frying pan, sauté onions in a bit of olive oil with garlic and a pinch of sage until caramelized.

- In blender or food processor, chop walnuts until very fine. Blend cooked brown rice in food processor and add a bit of water. Your mixture should be sticky and gooey.

- Put mixture into a bowl and add browned onions, bread crumbs, another pinch of sage, and sea salt to taste.

- Mix all ingredients together and make sure mixture will hold together. If mixture is too dry, add a bit more water; if too moist, you may need to add more bread crumbs. Form into patties.

- In a large frying pan with a touch of olive oil, brown patties on both sides over medium heat for a few minutes.

Yields 8 burgers.

NOTE

These burgers tend to be more mushy than dry, but they taste great and served with a tossed salad are perfect for lunch or dinner.

Hemp Burgers

Free of dairy products, wheat, yeast, corn, sugar, eggs, soy, nuts, and nightshades. If you use yeast-free bread, this is a yeast-free recipe.

- Wash hemp well in a fine sieve and place in a bowl. Bake sweet potato or squash with skin on in 350F oven or microwave until tender.

- In a skillet, brown onions in olive oil, add half amounts of sage, garlic, and salt. Add carrots, celery, and zucchini and sauté for 2 minutes with less than 1/4 cup (50 ml) water.

- Cut cooked sweet potato or squash in half, scoop out of the skin, and mash in the bowl with the hemp seeds. Add in sautéed onions, vegetables, and leftover spices and mix well with a fork. Add bread crumbs until you have a consistency of a burger that will hold together. If mixture is too dry, add a touch more water, or if too watery, add arrowroot. If you want a crunchy burger, add more bread crumbs. I use either spelt or barley bread for my bread crumbs and I simply toast the bread and then put in the blender or food processor to make crumbs.

- Form hemp mixture into burger patties (helpful hint: rub olive oil on your hands before you shape burgers).

- In a frying pan, lightly brown each side of burger, 2-3 minutes on each side.

Yields 8-10 burgers.

Ingredients

1/2 cup	unhulled hemp seeds, washed (125 ml)
1	medium-sized cooked buttercup squash or 2 large cooked sweet potatoes
1 1/2 cup	wheat-free bread crumbs (375 ml)
1	medium onion, chopped
1 tsp	sage (5 ml)
1 tsp	sea salt (5 ml)
	Handful fresh parsley, chopped
1/2 cup	carrot, grated (125 ml)
2	stalks celery, finely chopped
2	small zucchini, grated
1 tsp	arrowroot dissolved in 1 Tbsp (15 ml) cold water (optional) (5 ml)
2	cloves garlic, minced
	Water
	Oil for frying

DID YOU KNOW?
Hempseed is high in protein, containing a good balance of omega-3 and omega-6 essential fatty acids, as well as GLA, and has no cholesterol.

Bean and Rice Burgers

Free of dairy products, wheat, yeast, corn, sugar, eggs, soy, nuts, and nightshades. If you use yeast-free bread this is a yeast-free recipe.

Ingredients

1 cup	blackeyed peas (250 ml)
1/2 cup	uncooked white basmati rice (125 ml)
1/2-3/4 cup	wheat-free bread crumbs (125-175 ml)
1/4 tsp	sea salt (1 ml)
1/2 tsp	cumin (2 ml)
2 tsp	fresh ginger, grated (10 ml)
1	bunch green onions, chopped
2 tsp	olive oil (10 ml)
	Lettuce leaves
	Burger buns (optional)
	Water

- Rinse and soak beans. I usually soak them overnight and then rinse well before cooking. In a saucepan place 4 cups water with 1 cup of rinsed beans and bring to a boil. Reduce to simmer and cook for 1 1/2 hours or until beans are soft.

- Drain beans and rinse. Return cooked beans to the same pot and add uncooked basmati rice and 2 cups water. Stir in salt, cumin, ginger, and green onions and bring to a simmer and cook for at least 15 minutes or until rice is done. Stir frequently at the end. Mixture should be soft and well combined. Stir in bread crumbs, and when the mixture is cool enough to handle, form into patties.

- In a frying pan, add a little olive oil, just enough to cover the bottom of the pan, and cook patties for about 4 minutes on each side. Serve on lettuce leaves or burger buns if you can tolerate them.

- You can also add in some chopped celery when cooking the beans and rice, as it adds a bit of crunch to the burgers.

Yields 8 burgers.

NOTE
A ginger grater is a great tool to have in your kitchen.

Fillings for Spelt Wraps

Free of dairy products, wheat, yeast, corn, sugar, eggs, soy, nuts, and nightshades.

Ingredients

1 cup	kasha, rye berries or oat berries (250 ml)
1 cup	cabbage (250 ml)
1 cup	carrots (250 ml)
1	leek, shredded
2 tsp	fresh ginger, grated (10 ml)
	Sea salt to taste
	Olive oil
	Water
	Package of spelt wraps

- To cook oats, rye, or kasha, check front of cookbook for cooking directions.

- Shred cabbage, carrots, and leeks. In a frying pan with a bit of olive oil, sauté leeks for 2 minutes. Add in cabbage, carrots, sea salt, and ginger.
  Add 1/4 cup (50 ml) water and let simmer for 5-10 minutes, stirring frequently. Once done, add this mixture to cooked grain and mix well. You can add in some tamari if you can tolerate soy.

- Fill your wheat-free wraps and enjoy. I purchase my spelt wraps at my local health food store. They are yeast free and are delicious.

Yields 5 large wraps.

NOTE
You can also omit ginger and use different herbs depending on your allergies. Try parsley or basil, cumin or curry.

Rice Roll Ups

Free of dairy products, wheat, yeast, corn, sugar, eggs, soy, nightshades, and gluten.

Ingredients

1/4-1/2	cabbage, shredded
4	carrots, shredded
1 cup	fresh parsley, finely chopped (250 ml)
1 cup	bean sprouts (250 ml)
1	onion, diced
3-4 Tbsp	olive oil (45-60 ml)
1	package rice roll wrappers (look for them in your local Chinese food grocery; they tend to be cheaper there than in the health food store)
1 tsp	sage (5 ml)
1 tsp	summer savory (5 ml)
1 tsp	thyme (5 ml)
1	clove garlic, minced

- In a cast-iron frying pan, sauté chopped onions in olive oil until nicely browned. Add sage, savory, thyme and garlic at the end of browning onions to add flavour.

- In a separate bowl, mix chopped cabbage, carrots, parsley, bean sprouts, and half of the browned onions. Pour 2 tablespoons (30 ml) of olive oil over mixture and mix together. (Use your food processor to shred your cabbage, carrots, and parsley.)

- Into a deep pan, pour 1 inch of water and bring to boil, turn off, and remove from heat. Carefully dunk rice wrappers into water just so they get wet and become gooey. Remove wrappers from water and place on a plate. Be careful not to burn your fingers. (This is a delicate job and I try to use tongs and my fingers, but be careful not to rip the wrappers with the tongs.)

- With gooey rice wrapper on the plate, add a spoonful of cabbage mixture and fold wrapper sides in first and then roll so that it looks like a very thick egg roll. Place rolled rice wrap in a lightly oiled glass lasagna pan. Then top with almond gravy and cook in oven at 375F for about 10-15 minutes.

Yields 9-10 roll ups.

Almond Gravy

Ingredients

3/4 cup	almonds, ground (175 ml)
1	medium onion, chopped
2	cloves garlic, minced
1 tsp	sea salt (5 ml)
	Water or Soup Stock
1	broccoli, cut into bite-size pieces

- Steam broccoli for a few minutes. Don't overcook it, as it depletes all the nutrients.

- Cook onions in your frying pan until slightly caramel-ized. This gives the gravy a lovely flavour.

- Grind almonds in your food processor until relatively fine. Add cooked broccoli, 2-4 tablespoons (30-60 ml) of water, soup stock, or whichever liquid you wish to use. I tend to save the water I cooked the broccoli in and use that. Add garlic, sea salt, and cooked onion and mix well.

- Spread mixture over your rice roll ups and bake at 350F for 10-15 minutes until brown. Don't cook too long or it will dry out the rice wrappers.

DID YOU KNOW?

ALMONDS are probably the best all-around nut. Their fat content is less than most, about 60%, and the protein concentration is nearly 20%. The presence of 2-4% amygdalin, commonly known as Laetrile, has caused almonds to be considered as a cancer-preventing nut.

Salmon Croquettes

Free of dairy products, wheat, yeast, corn, sugar, eggs, soy, and nuts. If you use yeast-free bread this is a yeast-free recipe.

Ingredients

5-6	potatoes
1	medium onion, diced
1	can salmon (213 grams or 7.5 ounces)
3	sprigs fresh dill (optional)
	Handful fresh parsley, chopped (optional)
	Olive oil
1 cup	wheat-free bread crumbs (optional) (250 ml)
1	lemon

- Boil potatoes until soft and mash with leftover potato water or rice milk. Do not make mashed potatoes too watery, as you want your croquettes to stay together and not fall apart.

- In a frying pan, sauté onions until brown.

- In a bowl, mix salmon, mashed potatoes, dill, parsley, and browned onion. Add bread crumbs, or use a small amount of brown rice flour, arrowroot, or tapioca flour to help mixture stay together if it is too moist.

- Mix all ingredients together, and with your hands form into patties.

- In a frying pan with a little olive oil to cover the bottom of the pan, brown patties on medium high, approximately 3 minutes on each side. It is nice to serve them with a wedge of lemon.

- If you do not wish to fry the croquettes you can put them in the oven on a cookie sheet on the top rack to brown, but brush both sides with olive oil and bake at 375F. They do not need much time — just enough to brown. Do not overcook, as it will dry them out.

Yields 10 croquettes.

Ratatouille

Free of dairy products, wheat, yeast, corn, sugar, eggs, soy, nuts, and gluten.

- Sauté onions and garlic in olive oil, and let cook for a few minutes. Then add the rest of the cut-up vegetables and add enough olive oil to cover the bottom of the pan so that the vegetables will not burn.

- Cover, stir occasionally, and let simmer on low heat for about an hour and serve over favourite pasta or with rice.

Yields 4 cups (1 L).

Ingredients

1	eggplant, cut and cubed
1	medium zucchini, sliced
1	onion, diced
1	green pepper, diced
1	red pepper, diced
	Sea salt to taste
1 tsp	oregano (5 ml)
2	cloves garlic, minced
	Handful of fresh basil or 2 tsp (10 ml) dry basil
	Olive oil

Vegetarian Shepherd's Pie

Free of dairy products, wheat, yeast, corn, sugar, eggs, soy, nuts, and gluten.

Ingredients

1 cup	northern beans (250 ml)
1 cup	pinto beans (250 ml)
5-6	potatoes, sliced
1	medium onion, finely chopped
1/2 tsp	dry mustard (2 ml)
1 Tbsp	maple syrup (15 ml)
2	cloves garlic, minced
1 Tbsp	fresh ginger, grated (15 ml)
1 1/2 tsp	dried basil (7 ml)
1 1/2 tsp	dried thyme (7 ml)
2 Tbsp	fresh parsley (30 ml)
1 tsp	tarragon (5 ml)
2	stalks celery, diced
2	carrots, diced
1	bunch of kale, spinach, or swiss chard
2	medium zucchini, sliced
	Sunflower seeds (optional)

- To cook beans, bring to a boil, then simmer for 30 minutes, then rinse in cold water. Put beans back into pot with enough water to cover and cook on medium heat for 1 hour or until soft.

- In another pot, wash, peel, and boil potatoes to make mashed potatoes. You can use half sweet potatoes or even half turnip in with the white potatoes for a change. While boiling potatoes I put a sieve on top of the pot and steam kale, spinach, or swiss chard at the same time as boiling potatoes. It's a great way to steam vegetables and not use an extra pot. If you don't have a big sieve or steamer, you will have to steam greens separately.

- Mash potatoes however you wish. I mash them with a touch of olive oil and a bit of the potato water so they are moist. Add parsley and tarragon to taste.

- In a pan, lightly stir-fry zucchini, carrots, onions, and garlic in a little olive oil.

74

Vegetarian Shepherd's Pie

- In a glass lasagna pan layer beans on bottom, mix in mustard, maple syrup, basil, thyme, and ginger. Then add a layer of stir-fried veggies, a layer of kale or spinach, and top with mashed potatoes. You can sprinkle some sunflower seeds on top of the potatoes if you like.

- Broil for a few minutes in the oven to brown the top of the potatoes.

Yields 8 servings.

NOTE

Soak beans overnight, rinse many times. You can use a piece of Kombu when soaking to help eliminate the gaseous enzymes. Use 1 cup beans to 2 cups water for cooking.

For a less time-consuming recipe, you can use canned beans.

Beef Shepherd's Pie

Free of dairy products, wheat, yeast, corn, sugar, eggs, soy, nuts, and gluten.

Ingredients

2 lbs	lean ground beef (1 kg)
1	small onion, diced
	Olive oil
4	large potatoes (they can be white or sweet potatoes, or try half and half)
1	small bag of frozen peas
1 tsp	thyme (5 ml)
1/2 cup	water (125 ml)
2 tsp	cornstarch or arrowroot flour (diluted in 2 Tbsp [30 ml] cold water) (10 ml)
	Rice milk (optional)
	Sea salt and pepper to taste

- In a bit of olive oil, brown beef with onions, salt, pepper, and thyme. Once browned, add cornstarch mixture and let simmer for 1 minute, stir, and let gravy thicken.

- Boil potatoes in a pot and mash with some of the potato cooking water, or some rice milk.

- Place meat into a glass casserole dish, 9X9 inches. Add peas and top with mashed white or sweet potatoes. If you are using frozen peas, remember to cook them for a minute or so before adding them.

Yields 6 servings.

NOTE
If you wish to avoid corn, use arrowroot to thicken your gravy instead of cornstarch.

Lentil Shepherd's Pie

Free of dairy products, wheat, yeast, corn, sugar, eggs, soy, nuts, nightshades, and gluten.

Ingredients

1 cup	lentils (red or brown) (250 ml)
1	onion, diced
1	clove garlic
3	sweet potatoes, sliced
1	small bag frozen peas
2	carrots, sliced
2	bay leaves
1 tsp	tarragon (5 ml)
	Olive oil
	Sea salt
	Rice milk (optional)

- In a pot, cook 1 cup lentils with 3 cups water, bay leaf, and clove of garlic. I usually smash my garlic with a knife to open it up and let flavour out. Lentils take about 20 minutes to cook. When done, drain lentils, remove bay leaves, and mix garlic into lentils.

- Place lentils in the bottom of a casserole dish. Bring frozen peas to a boil and drain.

- Meanwhile, slice and cut up sweet potatoes and carrots and boil until soft. Mash sweet potatoes and carrots with leftover cooking water or a bit of rice milk. You can add salt, pepper, or margarine or whatever you can tolerate.

- In a frying pan, sauté and brown onions with a bit of tarragon or your choice of herbs. When done, spoon onions on top of lentils, followed by a layer of peas and then a layer of mashed sweet potato.

- Place in the oven and broil for a few minutes, just until the potatoes are lightly browned.

Yields 6 servings.

DID YOU KNOW?

Lentils are good for you, fast to cook, and do not need to be pre-soaked like beans.

Baked Beans

Free of dairy products, wheat, yeast, corn, sugar, eggs, soy, nuts, nightshades, and gluten.

Ingredients

2 cups	white navy beans (500 ml)
2 cups	pinto beans (500 ml)
2	medium onions, finely chopped
1 1/2 tsp	sea salt (7 ml)
2 tsp	lemon juice (10 ml)
2 tsp	dry mustard, or honey mustard if you can tolerate (10 ml)
2 Tbsp	maple syrup (30 ml)
1/2 cup	olive oil (125 ml)
1/2-1 cup	organic apple cider or apple juice (125-250 ml)
1 1/2 tsp	thyme (7 ml)
1/4 tsp	black pepper (1 ml)
2 1/2 tsp	summer savory (12 ml)
1/2-1 tsp	sage (2-5 ml)

- Soak beans overnight and rinse well. You can use a piece of kombu that has been rinsed when soaking your beans. It will help to eliminate the gaseous enzymes in the beans that cause flatulence. If you do not have kombu, don't worry, just rinse the beans a few times.

- Put the beans in a pot, cover them with cold filtered water and bring to a boil. Then let them simmer with lid on and leave for approximately 1 hour or until the beans are soft.

- Sauté onions in some olive oil with a pinch of sage and summer savory until onions are nicely brown.

- Place cooked beans, browned onions, and all other ingredients in a casserole dish and stir well. With lid on, bake beans for at least 1-2 hours, checking regularly, and stirring often. Beans should have some liquid in them. Bake at 325-350F for 2 hours, until beans are brown and creamy. Make sure there is liquid in the dish; if drying out, add more apple cider or a bit more oil to keep them moist.

Yields 10 cups.

Baked Beans

NOTE
Do not aDD saLt when cooking beans on the stove, as it wiLL take the beans Longer to cook. ALways aDD saLt near enD of cooking.

DID YOU kNOW?
That a Pot fuLL of beans is a Pot fuLL of nutrition! Rich in Protein, caLcium, PhosPhorus, anD iron, beans make a great meal.

Easy Beef or Lamb Stew

Free of dairy products, wheat, yeast, corn, sugar, eggs, soy, and nuts. This can be gluten- free if you use arrowroot instead of spelt flour.

Ingredients

1/2 cup	spelt flour (125 ml)
1/2 tsp	paprika (2 ml)
2 tsp	sea salt (10 ml)
	Olive oil
1	large onion, cut in quarters
1/2	turnip, diced
3-4	carrots, sliced
3-4	stalks celery, sliced
2	potatoes, diced (optional) or try sweet potato
1-2	cloves garlic, minced
1/2 cup	green beans (125 ml)
1-2	parsnips, sliced
2	bay leaves
	Water
2 lbs	Stewing beef or lamb stew pieces (1 kg)

- Mix spelt flour, paprika and salt together. Roll beef pieces in flour mixture and then coat with olive oil.

- Place the beef in a casserole dish or a clay baker if you have one. Bake uncovered for 25 minutes at 450F so that you singe the beef on all sides. Stir often. Once the beef is singed on both sides, scrape the sides of your dish so the singed meat is in the bottom of the dish. Add cut-up carrots, potatoes, turnip, parsnip, green beans, celery, and whatever other vegetable you like in your stew. Add salt, garlic, and other spices that you may wish. You can add a bay leaf or onion salt, whatever you can tolerate.

NOTE

I mix flour mixture in a tupperware container, add beef, seal, and shake to coat the beef.

For a gluten free recipe coat your beef or lamb with cornstarch. Use a little less if using cornstarch instead of spelt flour.

Easy Beef or Lamb Stew

- Mix 2 cups (500 ml) water with the leftover flour mixture that beef was rolled in and pour over beef and vegetables and cook at 325F for at least 2 hours. Stir once or twice, and if it is too dry add more water. Enjoy! It makes a great fall or winter meal.

  If you are using lamb, you can throw in some rosemary or oregano.

Yields 8 servings.

Stuffed Lamb

Free of dairy products, wheat, yeast, corn, sugar, eggs, nuts, and nightshades. If you use yeast-free bread this is a yeast-free recipe. If you use gluten-free bread crumbs it will be gluten-free.

Ingredients

3 lb	butterflied boneless leg of lamb (1.5 kg)
2	leeks, finely chopped
2 cups	spinach, washed and chopped (500 ml)
1/8 cup	fresh mint, chopped (25 ml)
1/8 cup	fresh rosemary, chopped (25 ml)
1/8 cup	fresh thyme, chopped (25 ml)
1/8 cup	fresh chives, chopped (25 ml)
1 cup	wheat-free bread crumbs (250 ml)
2 tsp	olive oil (10ml)
	Sea salt and pepper to taste

- Mix all ingredients except the lamb together in your food processor.

- I get my local butcher to butterfly the leg for me and open it up so I can stuff the lamb easily. Stuff leg of lamb and tie shut with string.

- Cook at 350F for as long as needed for the size of your roast. (Approximatively 25 minutes to the pound.)

Yields 5 servings.

Pineapple Meatballs

Free of dairy products, wheat, yeast, sugar, eggs, nuts, nightshades, and gluten.

Ingredients

Meatballs:

2 lbs	lean ground beef (1 kg)
1	medium onion, finely chopped
2	cloves garlic, minced
	Sea salt and pepper to taste
	Olive oil

Pineapple Sauce:

1 tsp	cornstarch (5 ml) mixed in 1 Tbsp (15 ml) cold water
1	can unsweetened pineapple chunks (14 fl oz. can) (398 ml)
1/2 cup	unsweetened pineapple juice (simply use the juice from the can of pineapple chunks) (125 ml)
1/3 cup	wheat-free soy sauce (tamari) (75 ml)
	Honey to taste

Meatballs:

- In a bowl, mix lean ground beef, salt, pepper, onion and garlic. Shape into balls and brown in olive oil in a skillet. Brown them quite quickly and sear them on all sides.

- Remove them and put them in a Dutch oven clay pot or casserole dish. Add pineapple sauce and bake slowly at 325F for 45 minutes.

- Serve over rice or with pasta.

Pineapple Sauce:

- Mix cornstarch with pineapple juice and add remaining ingredients to meatballs and cook.

Yields 20 meatballs.

NOTE
You can always use arrowroot powder or tapioca flour to thicken instead of cornstarch.

Caribou Meatloaf

Free of dairy products, wheat, yeast, corn, sugar, eggs, soy, nuts, nightshades and gluten.

Ingredients

1-1.5 lbs	ground caribou (.5-.7 kg)
1/4 cup	gluten-free rolled oats (50ml)
	Olive oil
2	cloves garlic, minced
1	small onion, chopped, Vidalia if you can get it
1	organic apple, diced, McIntosh or Spartan
1 tsp	oregano (5 ml)
1 tsp	salt (5 ml)
1 tsp	pepper (5 ml)

- Lightly coat your frying pan in olive oil and caramelize your onions in minced garlic. Towards the end of cooking, add in cut-up apple, oregano, salt, and pepper. Cook for a few minutes, then remove from heat and let cool.

- In a bowl, mix ground caribou and rolled oats together. Then add in cooked onion and apple mixture and mix all together.

- Place meat mixture in a meatloaf pan and let sit in your fridge for a couple of hours. (I make my meatloaf in the morning and let it sit in the fridge all day; it seems to enhance the flavours.)

- Cook meatloaf for approximately 1 hour at 350-375F.

Slice and enjoy. Serve with Chutney.

Yields 1 loaf or 4 servings.

NOTE
You can use caribou, venison, bison, or beef for this meatloaf.

Chutney

Free of dairy products, wheat, yeast, corn, sugar, eggs, soy, nuts, nighshades, and gluten.

- In a small pot, caramelize your onion in some apple juice, and add in diced apple, ginger, and blueberries. Mix and add a bit more apple juice if too dry.

- If you want, you can add some walnuts, but I like it as is.

  Serve on top of meatloaf.

Yields 1 cup (250 ml).

Ingredients

1	McIntosh apple, diced
1/4	onion, diced, Vidalia if you can get it (they have such a lovely flavour)
2 Tbsp	organic apple juice (30 ml)
1 Tbsp	fresh ginger, grated (15 ml)
1	small garlic clove, minced (optional)
1/2 cup	blueberries (125 ml)

Beef Stir Fry Wrapped in Lettuce Leaves

Free of dairy products, wheat, yeast, corn, sugar, eggs, soy, nuts, and gluten.

Ingredients

1.5 lbs	sirloin steak, cut into small lengthwise strips (.7 kg)
1-2	cloves garlic, minced
1-2 tsp	fresh ginger, grated (5-10 ml)
1	medium onion, diced
2	carrots, diced
2-3	celery stalks, diced
	Red or green pepper, diced (optional)
	Olive oil
	Iceberg or romaine lettuce
	Bean sprouts
	Toasted sesame oil

- Try to remove outer layers of lettuce leaves in full. Wash and let drip dry.

- In a wok, pour enough olive oil to cover bottom. Turn on high and cook strips of beef with garlic.
  Do not fully cook. Take meat out of wok and place in a bowl. Then cook onions in the leftover oil, as the meat juice will help to brown the onions and give them more flavour. Add diced carrots, peppers, zucchini, or any other vegetable you desire and cook until the veggies are almost done (I like mine still a bit crispy, so it does not take long). When you are cooking with a wok, you need to be continuously stirring so that the food does not burn. Add the beef to finish cooking, then grated ginger, diced celery, and sprouts. At this time you can add a few drops of toasted sesame oil, as it adds a lovely flavour to your beef.

- Spoon mixture into lettuce leaves, roll, and eat.

NOTE
Another option is to use sirloin bison meat in this recipe. Bison is high in iron and low in fat.

Beef Stir Fry Wrapped in Lettuce Leaves

- You can also cook some organic rice and add a bit into the lettuce leaves as well; or if you have the energy and you wish to roll the beef in cabbage rolls, simply blanch cabbage leaves first. I like the lettuce leaf option, as it is quick and easy and a change from regular stir-fry.

- If beef is a problem, replace with organic chicken, pork, or even shrimp. If you are a vegetarian, simply enjoy stir-fried veggies with rice in your lettuce leaves, or add in some TVP (textured vegetable protein) strips. I use tofu.

Yields 2 servings.

DID YOU KNOW?
That there are hundreds of varieties of lettuce grown around the world, and that lettuce is rich in calcium, iron, and vitamins A and C.

Stuffed Grape Leaves

Free of dairy products, wheat, yeast, corn, sugar, eggs, soy, nuts, nightshades, and gluten.

Ingredients

1	small jar grape leaves
1	medium onion, ½ finely chopped
1	leek, finely chopped
12	snow peas, chopped
1 cup	cooked brown rice (250ml)
½ cup	carrot, finely chopped (125 ml)
2	cloves garlic, minced
1	lemon, squeezed
	Olive oil
1 cup	brown lentils (250 ml)
1 tsp	summer savoury (5ml)
2	bay leaves
	Sea salt to taste

- Cook brown lentils in a pot of water with half an onion, 2 bay leaves, and a pinch of savoury. Cook until soft, approximately 20 minutes. Remove bay leaves and onion, then take cooked brown lentils and mix in a food processor or blender until it has the consistency of a sauce.

- In a pan, sauté onion, leek, and carrot in olive oil and garlic for 3 minutes. Near the end of cooking, add cooked rice, snow peas, salt, and lemon juice.

- Spread out grape leaves onto a plate and put a small amount of rice mixture inside each one. Roll leaves and place in a lightly greased 9x13 inch glass baking dish. Once rolled and placed in dish, cover with the lentil mixture.

- Bake at 350F for about 20 minutes. Be careful not to cook too long, or they will dry out.

Yields 20 rolls.

Tuna and Pasta

Free of dairy products, wheat, yeast, corn, sugar, eggs, soy, and nuts. This can be gluten free if you use rice, quinoa, or buckwheat pasta.

- In a cast-iron pan, cook onions, peppers, broccoli, ginger, and celery in some olive oil over medium heat. When vegetables are done, add the can of drained tuna to the vegetables. Stir for a few minutes so that the tuna gets warmed.

- In separate pot, cook wheat-free pasta. In a bowl, toss stir-fried vegetables and tuna with the hot pasta and enjoy.

There are so many wheat-free pastas these days, the options are endless. Kamut, spelt, quinoa, corn, brown rice, or mung bean. Whether you mix your pasta with veggies, beef, or fish, it makes a great meal.

Yields 2 servings.

Ingredients

1	can tuna, packed in water
1	bunch green onions, diced
	Olive oil
1/2	red or green pepper, sliced (optional)
1	stalk celery, sliced
	Half a broccoli, cut into bite-sized pieces
	Fresh ginger, grated (if you cannot tolerate ginger, use garlic or any other herb you like)
2 cups	wheat-free pasta (kamut, spelt, rice, or quinoa pasta) (500 ml)

DID YOU KNOW?

Tuna is part of the mackerel family and is the most popular fish used for canning today. There are numerous varieties of tuna. The best known is albacore, and is packed in either water or oil. The latter contains more calories.

Sweet and Sour Chicken

Free of dairy products, wheat, yeast, corn, sugar, eggs, soy, nuts, and gluten.

Ingredients

2	pieces boneless, skinless chicken breast, cut into bite-sized pieces
1	onion, chopped
1 cup	celery, chopped (250 ml)
1 cup	carrots, chopped (250 ml)
1/2	red pepper, chopped

Sauce:

1 cup	unsweetened pineapple juice (250 ml)
1 Tbsp	apple cider vinegar (15 ml)
1 Tbsp	arrowroot powder or cornstarch (15 ml)
1/4 cup	water (50 ml)
	Olive oil
1 Tbsp	tomato paste (optional) (15 ml)

- In a frying pan with enough oil to cover bottom of pan, cook chicken over low to medium heat, stirring frequently, for approx. 10 minutes. Remove chicken and set aside.

- In a frying pan, sauté onions for a few minutes in a little olive oil or use a little water or vegetable stock. Add chopped celery, carrots, red pepper, and water and cook over medium heat for 10 minutes. Then add the chicken pieces.

- In a separate bowl, mix sauce ingredients and pour over chicken, add vegetables and simmer for a few minutes.

Serve with a mixed salad or steamed veggies.

Yields 2 servings.

Simple Chicken Dinner

Free of dairy products, wheat, yeast, corn, sugar, eggs, soy, nuts, and gluten.

Ingredients

- In a glass oven dish, brush bottom with olive oil so chicken will not burn or stick.

- Place frozen chicken, onions, peppers, salt, and pepper in a glass dish. Place aluminum foil over pan and put in oven at 400F for 1 hour or until done. Cooking the chicken frozen makes a lovely, juicy chicken and it is so easy, no waiting for the chicken to defrost.

  Remove foil at the end to brown the chicken skin if you like.

  Serve with steamed veggies and a salad, and you have a wonderful fast, easy meal.

Yields 2 servings.

2	large frozen organic or grain-fed chicken breasts or legs
2	medium onions, chopped in quarters
1	red pepper, chopped in quarters
1	green pepper, chopped in quarters
	Sea salt and pepper to taste
	Olive oil

Garlic Shrimp with Lime

Free of dairy products, wheat, yeast, corn, sugar, eggs, soy, nuts, nightshades, and gluten.

Ingredients

18	uncooked shrimp
3 Tbsp	olive oil, margarine or butter (45ml)
3-4	cloves garlic, minced
2	limes
	Handful fresh parsley, finely chopped

- Thaw shrimp if frozen; de-vein if not done.

- In a large frying pan, melt butter or margarine with garlic over medium heat. Add juice of 1 lime, salt, and pepper.

- Place shrimp in pan and cook for a few minutes until they are a lovely pink colour. Sprinkle more lime juice and simmer.

- Sprinkle fresh parsley on shrimp and serve with a salad or over rice. Delicious.

  I get my fresh shrimp at either my local fish store or I buy a bag of large, uncooked, de-veined Tiger shrimp at my local grocery store.

Yields 2 servings.

Barbequed Red Snapper

Free of dairy products, wheat, yeast, corn, sugar, eggs, soy, nuts, and gluten.

Ingredients

2	fresh red snapper fillets (or any fresh fish fillets of your choice)
1	large red pepper, sliced
1/4 cup	water or soup stock (50 ml)
2 Tbsp	fresh ginger, grated (30 ml)
1/2	lemon, juiced, or 1/4 tsp (1 ml) wine vinegar
	Sea salt to taste

- Slice red pepper in half and roast on barbeque grill or on a baking sheet under your broiler until skin is blackened.

- Place charred pepper in brown paper bag or cover with a linen tea towel and let sit 10 minutes. This will trap the steam and make it easier to remove the blackened skin.

- Scrape blackened skin off pepper and discard any seeds.

- In a blender or food processor, purée pepper with water, vinegar, salt, and ginger.

- Barbeque snapper fillets for about 4 minutes on each side or until fish is done.

Serve with purée over top of filets.

Yields 2 servings.

You know, the less you do to fish, the better. I love it pan-fried in a little olive oil with a squirt of lemon. It satisfies without filling you and digests so easily. These days we can get so many types of fish that the options are endless. Yes, some are more expensive than others but worth treating yourself to once in awhile.

BBQ Fish Fillets

Free of dairy products, wheat, yeast, corn, sugar, eggs, soy, nuts, and gluten.

Ingredients

2	fish fillets, haddock, sole, tuna, or whatever your preference
2	avocados
2	mangoes
1 Tbsp	fresh lemon juice (15 ml)
2	small cucumbers
2 Tbsp	olive oil (30 ml)
	Jasmine rice or basmati rice

Dressing:

1/3 cup	fresh lemon juice (75 ml)
2 Tbsp	sweet chili sauce (30 ml)

If you cannot have chili sauce, use:

1	red pepper, finely chopped with 3 sliced green onions
1 Tbsp	fresh chives, chopped (15 ml)
	Sea salt and pepper to taste

- Halve and peel avocados and cut into slices. Place in a bowl and sprinkle lemon juice over them so they don't turn brown.

- Peel mangoes and slice thinly. Set aside in a bowl.

- Wash cucumbers and with a peeler, peel off some strips of cucumber lengthwise to form long ribbons.

- To make the dressing, combine lemon juice, chili sauce, chopped peppers, and chives in a jar and shake well.

- Brush fish fillets with olive oil, lemon juice, salt, and pepper. Barbeque fillets until done, about 4 minutes on each side; or pan fry.

To serve, place fish fillets on plate and arrange mango, avocado, and cucumber slices over fish and pour dressing over top. Serve with basmati or jasmine rice or with a tossed salad.

Yields 2 servings.

Fish Fingers

Free of dairy products, wheat, yeast, corn, sugar, eggs, soy, and nightshades. If you use the soy milk, this recipe will not be soy free. For a gluten free option use either millet, rice or chickpea flour

- Dip fish fillets into milk, roll in flour, and then coat with sesame seeds or almonds.

- Place coated fish in a lightly greased glass baking dish and bake fish in a moderate 350F oven until done, for approximately 30 minutes, depending on thickness of fish.

Ingredients

Thick fish fillets
(your choice of fish)

Allowable flour (spelt, barley, oat, millet, rice, chickpea)

Nut milk, rice milk, or soy milk

Sesame seeds or finely ground almonds

Olive oil

Vegetarian Tourtière

Free of dairy products, wheat, yeast, corn, sugar, eggs, soy, nuts, and nightshades.

Ingredients

Crust:

6 cups	spelt flour (1.5 L)
2 tsp	sea salt (10 ml)
1 1/3 cup	oil (325 ml)
1 cup	very hot water (250 ml)

Crust:

- In a mixing bowl, place dry ingredients and fluff with a whisk. Add wet ingredients and stir with a fork. This recipe makes a very oily dough and enough for three pies. Divide dough into 6 equal balls. Roll out dough between sheets of waxed paper with a rolling pin.

- Line pie shells with pastry, add filling, and cover with the top crust.

Vegetarian Tourtière

Ingredients

Filling:

4	large onions, diced
7	cloves garlic, minced
1/2 cup	olive oil (or enough to generously cover the bottom of your pot) (125 ml)
1/2 cup	spelt flour (125 ml)
3 Tbsp	summer savoury (45 ml)
3/4 tsp	allspice (3 ml)
3/4 tsp	cloves (3 ml)
3/4 tsp	cinnamon (3 ml)
3/4 tsp	nutmeg (3 ml)
3/4 tsp	black pepper (3 ml)
1 Tbsp	sea salt (15 ml)
1 1/2 cups	warm water (375 ml)

Cooked grains:

2 cups	cooked brown rice (500 ml)
2 cups	cooked millet (500 ml)
2 cups	cooked barley (500 ml)
4 cups	cooked beans (pinto beans are good in this recipe; mash them up a bit) (1 L)

Filling:

- In a large pan, sauté onions and garlic in olive oil until transparent. Then add spelt flour and continue to cook for 2 minutes on medium heat, stirring constantly. Add water, herbs, and sea salt. Stir until thick.

- Turn off heat and add cooked grains and mashed beans. Mix all ingredients well and fill pie shells. Cover with top crust and cut slits into top of dough with a knife, and bake for 45 minutes in 350F oven.

This recipe yields 3 pies and they freeze well.

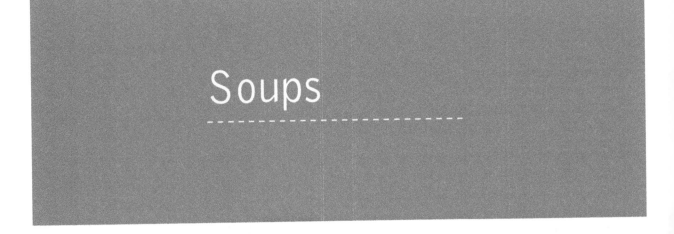

Soups

100   Beef, Chicken, or Vegetable Stock

101   Red Lentil Sweet Potato Soup

102   Parsnip Soup

103   Millet Vegetable Soup

104   Creamy Cauliflower Soup

105   Carrot Soup

106   Leek and Potato Soup

107   Split Pea Soup

108   Veggie Barley Soup

109   Spinach and Pear Soup

110   Cream of Broccoli Soup

111   Quinoa Soup

112   Zucchini Soup

113   Borscht

Beef, Chicken, or Vegetable Stock

Ask your local butcher for some beef marrow bones.

In a pot, place enough water to cover bones, and boil up beef bones for about 30 minutes. You can add a cut-up onion, carrots, celery, and fresh parsley as well to the water; this will make you a nice, flavourful stock.

If you have the time and the energy, place your beef bones on a baking sheet and brown in the oven at 350F for about 15 minutes. This will enhance their flavour before you boil them. After you have boiled your bones, place boiled liquid in a bowl in the refrigerator and, once cooled, skim off the fat. Throw out beef bones or give them to your dog as a treat. Use liquid for a beef soup stock.

For a basic chicken stock, simply take the carcass from your cooked chicken the night before and boil it in a pot with water, an onion, and some celery stalks. Again pour liquid into a bowl and place in the refrig-erator. Skim off excess fat and use liquid as stock.

For a basic vegetable stock, boil an onion, organic carrot peels, celery hearts and tops, a few slices of burdock, and any other naturally sweet vegetable that you have around the house. I save odds and ends of vegetables throughout the week in a container. I also save boiled water from vegetables that I have cooked that week, as it makes good soup stock as well. Try to keep boiled veggie water in a glass jar in the fridge so that when you want to make soup it is there.

The soup recipes that are in this book can all be made without soup stock and with only water. I wanted easy, tasty soup recipes for people to be able to make who are either not able to take the time to make homemade soups or do not have the energy.

I used to avoid making soups for the simple reason that I did not have the energy to make soup stock before making my soups. Now I can make quick, yummy soups and have them on hand for my lunches.

These soup recipes are basic so that you can play with the recipes. You can add more herbs and seasonings if you can tolerate them, or even start from scratch and make your own soup stock. Throw in some lentils or beans to make the soup more of a stew, or purée it for creamier textures. It is all up to you.

Red Lentil Sweet Potato Soup

Free of dairy products, wheat, yeast, corn, sugar, eggs, soy, nuts, nightshades, and gluten.

I love this recipe, as it is quick, easy to make, and very tasty. I also found that when I was first avoiding certain foods, I could tolerate all these ingredients.

- Wash lentils and discard any foreign objects. If you buy organic red lentils, you sometimes find little rocks in with them.

- In a soup pot, sauté onion or leek in oil for 5 minutes. Add cut-up sweet potatoes, carrots, salt, and cumin, and cook in the oil for a few minutes. Add lentils with water.

- Simmer soup on low for 30 minutes, stirring occasionally. Purée soup in your food processor, or use a hand-held mixer. This makes quite a thick soup.

Ingredients

	olive oil
1 cup	red lentils (250 ml)
4-5 cups	water (1-1.25 L)
3	large carrots, sliced
1	medium onion, diced, or 1 leek, finely chopped
1	large sweet potato, sliced
1 tsp	sea salt (5 ml)
1 tsp	cumin (5 ml)

NOTE

A hand-held mixer is a great tool to have in your kitchen. I use mine all the time. You can adapt this soup and instead of using sweet potato you can use white potatoes or 1 cup of wild rice. If you use rice, you may need to add a bit more water when cooking. I would not purée the soup if using rice. You can also use freshly grated ginger instead of cumin as your seasoning.

Parsnip Soup

Free of dairy products, wheat, yeast, corn, sugar, eggs, soy, nuts, and gluten.

Ingredients

3 Tbsp	olive oil (45 ml)
2 1/2 cups	parsnips, peeled and diced (625 ml)
	Half of a large butternut squash, peeled and diced
1	small onion, diced
2	large potatoes, peeled and diced
6	green onions, sliced
3	stalks celery, diced
2	cloves garlic, minced
1 tsp	dried sage (5 ml)
2 tsp	sea salt (10 ml)
1/2 tsp	pepper (2 ml)
4-6 cups	water (1-1.5 L)

- Chop green onions and set aside.

- Over medium-high heat, sauté onion and garlic in olive oil until onions are translucent.

- Add all vegetables except green onions and stir continuously for 1 minute.

- Add water, sage, salt, and pepper and let simmer for about 25 minutes.

- Add green onions and let sit for a few minutes.

  Blend or purée soup.

Yields 8 cups (2 L).

DID YOU KNOW?
That Europeans brought the parsnip to the United States in the early 1600s? Parsnips have a lovely, sweet flavour to them and contain vitamin C and iron.

Millet Vegetable Soup

Free of dairy products, wheat, yeast, corn, sugar, eggs, soy, nuts, nightshades, and gluten.

This soup is delicious and good for you. Millet is full of nutrients and easy to digest.

- In a large soup pot, cover bottom of pot with olive oil and sauté onions over medium high heat. Let your onions sweat for about 2 minutes.

- Add cabbage, carrots, squash, turnip, garlic, and a touch more olive oil and stir frequently. You want to sauté the vegetables for a few minutes; this will bring out their flavour.

- Add rinsed millet (always rinse your millet to remove dirt and dust) and stir for 30 seconds.

- Add water and all seasonings and bring to a boil and then let simmer for 30 minutes.

- Remove bay leaves and enjoy.

Yields 12 cups (3 L).

DID YOU KNOW?
Millet is gluten free and is a great grain to use to thicken soups, stews, and casseroles.

Ingredients

	Olive oil
1 cup	millet (250 ml)
1	butternut squash, peeled and cubed
1/2 cup	shredded cabbage (125 ml)
4	carrots, sliced
1/2	turnip, diced into bite-size pieces
1	medium red onion, diced
2	cloves garlic, minced
1 cup	fresh parsley, chopped (250 ml)
2 tsp	basil (10 ml)
1 tsp	celery seed (5 ml)
1 tsp	pepper (5 ml)
1-2 tsp	sea salt (5-10 ml)
3	bay leaves
6-7 cups	water (1.5-1.75 L)

Creamy Cauliflower Soup

Free of dairy products, wheat, yeast, corn, sugar, eggs, soy, nuts, nightshades, and gluten.

Ingredients

3 Tbsp	olive oil (45 ml)
1	medium onion, chopped
3	cloves garlic, minced
3	stalks celery, chopped
1	medium cauliflower, chopped into bite-size pieces
1/2 cup	millet or quinoa, rinsed (125 ml)
4 cups	water or vegetable stock (1 L)
	Handful fresh parsley or spinach, chopped
1 tsp	sea salt (5 ml)
1/2 tsp	pepper (2 ml)
1/2 tsp	dried thyme (2 ml)
1 tsp	basil (5 ml)
1/4 tsp	dry mustard (1 ml)
2	bay leaves

- In a soup pot, sauté onions in a little olive oil for about 2 minutes. Let your onions sweat and become translucent.

- Add cauliflower, celery, garlic, and a touch more olive oil if you need it. On medium high, cook vegetables for about 3 minutes. Stir often; you want your veggies to sweat. Then add millet or quinoa and stir for 30 seconds. Add water or vegetable stock, enough to cover all the vegetables and millet handsomely, and bring to a boil.

- Add seasonings, lower heat, and simmer for 20-25 minutes, until cauliflower is cooked. Add parsley or spinach and using a handheld blender, blend until smooth.

Yields 8 cups (2 L).

DID YOU KNOW?
According to Mark Twain, "cauliflower is nothing but cabbage with a college education." Known as a cruciferous vegetable, it is high in vitamin C.

Carrot Soup

Free of dairy products, wheat, yeast, corn, sugar, eggs, soy, nuts, nightshades, and gluten.

- In a soup pot, sauté onion in oil for 2 minutes on medium heat; do not brown. Let the onions sweat and get transparent. Add carrots and ginger and a touch more olive oil. Stir frequently for 1 minute.
  Add vegetable stock or water and bring to a boil.

- Add salt, pepper, and thyme and simmer gently for 20 minutes or until the carrots are tender.

- Purée the soup in a blender or food processor or use a hand-held blender.

  Garnish with parsley or green onions if you like.

  Options: You can also add in parsley at the end of cooking. Some cooked millet also makes this soup very tasty.

Yields 4 cups (1 L).

Ingredients

3 Tbsp	olive oil (45 ml)
4 cups	carrots, sliced (1 L)
1	medium onion, chopped
2 tsp	fresh ginger, grated (more if you like the taste of ginger) (10 ml)
4 cups	water or vegetable stock (1 L)
1/4 tsp	thyme (optional) (1 ml)
	Handful fresh parsley, chopped
1	bunch of green onions (4 green onions, chopped)
	Sea salt and pepper to taste

NOTE

A great kitchen tool is a ginger grater. Mine is ceramic and is in the shape of a pineapple. It has bumps all over it and you simply rub the fresh ginger over the bumps and voila, grated ginger.

You can also buy little stainless steel graters. A must in the kitchen, especially if you like fresh ginger.

Leek and Potato Soup

Ingredients

Free of dairy products, wheat, yeast, corn, sugar, eggs, soy, nuts, and gluten.

3 Tbsp	olive oil (45 ml)
4	leeks, washed well and sliced
7-8	medium potatoes, peeled and diced
7-8 cups	water or vegetable stock (1.75-2 L)
	Sea salt and pepper to taste
	Parsley, chives, or watercress to garnish

- In a soup pot, sauté leeks and potatoes very gently in oil on medium heat for 3 minutes and stir often. Add water or stock and simmer for 25 minutes, until potatoes are tender.

- Add handful of parsley, purée in blender, and serve. Add salt, pepper, and whichever herbs you can tolerate to taste.

  I personally love to sprinkle cut, fresh chives on top of my potato soup.

Yields 9 cups (2.25 L).

DID YOU KNOW?
The leek is related to both garlic and onion, though its flavour is milder and more subtle.

When purchasing leeks, choose those with crisp, brightly coloured leaves.

Split Pea Soup

Free of dairy products, wheat, yeast, corn, sugar, eggs, soy, nuts, nightshades, and gluten. Paprika is from the nightshade family so if you want to avoid nightshades in your diet, omit the paprika.

Ingredients

4 Tbsp	olive oil (60 ml)
2 cups	split peas, rinsed well and drained (500 ml)
4	carrots, peeled and diced
4	stalks celery, sliced
1/2 cup	turnip, diced, or 1/2 cup cooked squash (125 ml)
1 1/2 tsp	thyme (7 ml)
1 1/2 tsp	basil (7 ml)
1	medium onion, finely chopped
1 tsp	dry mustard (5 ml)
1 1/2 tsp	sea salt (7 ml)
1 tsp	pepper (5 ml)
2	cloves garlic, minced
1 tsp	fresh grated ginger (5 ml)
1 tsp	paprika (optional) (5 ml)
5 cups	water (1.25 L)
	Handful fresh parsley, chopped

- In a large soup pot, sauté onions in olive oil, approx. 3 minutes.

- Once sautéed, add split peas and stir frequently for another 4 minutes. This allows the flavour of the split peas to come out. Add water, 1/2 teaspoon (2 ml) thyme, 1/2 teaspoon (2 ml) basil, and some fresh parsley.

- Let split peas simmer on low heat for 35 minutes with lid on.

- Add chopped celery, carrots, turnip, the rest of the basil and thyme, dry mustard, sea salt, pepper, crushed garlic, grated ginger, and paprika and let simmer for another 20 minutes with lid off.

- Purée soup if you like. This makes a lovely, thick soup.

  Another option for this soup is to add cooked wild rice at the end of cooking.

Yields 8 cups (2 L).

Veggie Barley Soup

Free of dairy products, wheat, yeast, corn, sugar, eggs, soy, and nuts.

Ingredients

3 Tbsp	olive oil (45 ml)
1	medium onion, chopped
3/4 cup	pearl barley (175 ml)
9 cups	water or soup stock (2.25 L)
2	bay leaves
4	large potatoes, diced
5	carrots, diced
1 cup	frozen green beans (250 ml)
1/2	turnip, diced
1/4 cup	fresh parsley, chopped (50 ml)
	Sea salt and pepper to taste

- In a soup pot with a little olive oil, cook onions until soft.

- Add barley and cook for 1 minute, stirring frequently.

- Add water, bay leaves, and pepper and bring to a boil.

- Reduce heat and let simmer for 1 hour.

- Then add potatoes, carrots, turnip, and salt and return to a boil and then simmer again on low for 30 minutes. Stir occasionally.

- Add green beans in the last 5 minutes of cooking.

  Discard bay leaves, add parsley, and serve. This makes a lovely, chunky, thick soup.

Yields 10 cups (2.5 L).

DID YOU KNOW?
Barley dates back to the Stone Age and has been used in dishes from cereal to breads to soups, one of the more well known of which is Scotch Broth.

Spinach and Pear Soup

Free of dairy products, wheat, yeast, corn, sugar, eggs, soy, nuts, nightshades, and gluten.

- In a large soup pot, sauté onions in olive oil for a few minutes. Add diced carrots and sauté for another few minutes.

- Add in rice and stir for 1 minute, then add pears, garlic, spices, bay leaves, water, and juice, and bring to a simmer.

- Cover and simmer for 15 minutes or until rice is done. Remove bay leaves and stir in chopped spinach. Add apple juice or more water if needed. If you are not using apple juice, you will have to add more water. At this point, you can add a couple dashes of toasted sesame oil if you like, as it gives the soup a lovely flavour.

- Simmer for another 3 minutes and then blend your soup.

Yields 8 cups (2 L).

DID YOU KNOW?
That spinach is "POWER PACKED," as Popeye would say, with vitamins A and C, and contains oxalic acid, which gives it that slightly bitter taste.

Soups

Ingredients

3 Tbsp	olive oil (45 ml)
1 cup	sushi rice, or long-grain white rice (250 ml)
1	medium onion, diced
4	bay leaves
1 tsp	cumin (5 ml)
3	large carrots, sliced
2	pears, cored and cut into small pieces
2	cloves garlic, minced
1 tsp	sesame oil (5 ml)
1	large bunch spinach, or package of spinach, washed and chopped
4-5 cups	water (1-1.25 L)
1 cup	apple juice (optional) (250 ml)
	A couple dashes toasted sesame oil (optional)
	Sea salt and pepper to taste

Cream of Broccoli soup

Free of dairy products, wheat, yeast, corn, sugar, eggs, soy, nuts, nightshades, and gluten.

Ingredients

3 Tbsp	olive oil (45 ml)
1	bunch broccoli, cut into small pieces, stalk included
1	medium onion, chopped
6-7 cups	water (1.5-1.75 L)
1 tsp	sea salt (5 ml)
1/2 tsp	pepper (2 ml)
2	cloves garlic, minced
3	stalks celery, chopped
1/2 cup	millet, washed (125 ml)
1 cup	rice milk (250 ml)
1 tsp	organic herbal salt (5 ml)
	Handful of fresh parsley, chopped

- Cut broccoli into small flowerets, including stems, which have been peeled and chopped.

- In a large soup pot, use a little olive oil to cover the bottom of the pan. Sauté onions on medium-high heat until they are transparent, approximately 2 minutes. At this time, add garlic and all cut-up vegetables except parsley, and stir constantly for 2 minutes.

- Add millet and stir for another minute. Be careful not to let millet stick or burn.

- Add water, salt, pepper, and herbal salt. Bring to a boil and then simmer for at least 25 minutes until millet is cooked.

- Turn off heat and add chopped parsley and rice milk and blend with hand blender.

  When you are ready to serve your soup, it is nice to squeeze some fresh lemon juice into it, as it brings out the flavour of the soup.

Yields 9 cups (2.25 L).

NOTE

Remember to always wash your millet before cooking as it can be dirty. You can add whatever seasoning you like to this soup. I buy organic herbal salt, which is a lovely seasoning to use in this recipe. It is a mixture of mineral salt, carrots, parsley, celery, basil, dill, leeks, and onions. Look for it in your local health food store.

Quinoa Soup

Free of dairy products, wheat, yeast, corn, sugar, eggs, soy, nuts, nightshades, and gluten.

- In a pot, sauté onions, carrots, and garlic in a small amount of olive oil.

- Add water, quinoa, and parsley.

- Bring to a boil and then simmer for about 20 minutes.

  This soup can be as simple as you like. Sometimes I just add whatever vegetables I have in the fridge — carrots or beans or celery.

  Quinoa is very soothing and good for the stomach when you are not feeling that well.

Yields 5 cups (1.25 L).

Ingredients

3 Tbsp	olive oil (45 ml)
1/2 cup	quinoa, rinsed (125 ml)
4 cups	water (1 L)
1/2	small onion, chopped
3	carrots, chopped
2	stalks celery, chopped
1/2	bag spinach, chopped (optional)
2	small cloves garlic, minced
	Sea salt and pepper to taste
	Handful fresh parsley, chopped

DID YOU KNOW?

That quinoa is considered a complete protein, as it contains all eight essential amino acids. It is also higher in unsaturated fats and lower in carbohydrates than most other grains and is full of nutrients.

Zucchini Soup

Free of dairy products, wheat, yeast, corn, sugar, eggs, soy, nuts, nightshades, and gluten.

Ingredients

	Olive oil
6 cups	zucchini, diced (approx. 3 large zucchini) (1.5 L)
1	medium onion, diced
2	cloves garlic, minced
3-4 cups	water or vegetable soup stock (750 ml-1 L)
1 tsp	basil (5 ml)
1 tsp	oregano (5 ml)
1 tsp	sea salt (5 ml)
1/2 tsp	pepper (2 ml)
1 can	beans – navy, lima, or northern beans (14 fl oz.-398 ml)
	Handful parsley or watercress to garnish (optional)

- Cut zucchini into small chunks. In a soup pot, heat oil and add onions and cook until soft, approximately 2 minutes.

- Add zucchini and garlic and cook, stirring frequently, for 2 minutes. Add soup stock or water, basil, oregano, salt, and pepper, and simmer for 15 minutes until zucchini is soft.

- Add canned beans and parsley and purée with hand-held blender.

You can serve this soup hot or cold.

Yields 8 cups (2 L).

DID YOU KNOW?
That zucchini is in fact a summer squash.

Borscht

Free of dairy products, wheat, yeast, corn, sugar, eggs, soy, nuts, nightshades, and gluten.

- Wash, peel, and cut beets into small pieces. Take off beet leaves, wash, and cut into pieces as well.

- Bring water to a boil in a pot and add beets and beet greens and boil for a few minutes.

- Then add the rest of the ingredients except for parsley, dill, and radishes and simmer for 40 minutes until all vegetables are cooked. Add dill, parsley, radishes, and a bit of lemon juice at the end.

  I like this soup, as the borscht that I have always had in restaurants tastes too much of vinegar.
  By using only a bit of lemon juice, you have a lovely soup that tastes of beets instead of vinegar.

Yields 12 cups (3 L).

NOTE

options for this soup are that you can add some diced zucchini if you are serving it hot, or slice a couple of radishes and add them if you are serving it cold.

Ingredients

1-2	bunches of beets, peeled and chopped
1-2	bunch beet greens, chopped
1	bunch green onions, chopped
3	carrots, diced
1/2 cup	green or red cabbage, shredded (125 ml)
3	stalks celery, diced
2 Tbsp	lemon juice (30 ml)
1	clove garlic, minced
3 Tbsp	fresh parsley, finely chopped (45 ml)
	Handful of fresh dill, finely chopped
11-12 cups	water or vegetable soup stock (2.75-3 L)
1	zucchini, diced (optional)
2-3	radishes, sliced (optional)
	Sea salt to taste

Salads and

Dressings

116   Quinoa Salad

117   Sweet Potato Salad

118   Potato Salad

119   Fruit Salad

120   Good Ol' Fashioned Cabbage Salad

121   Waldorf Salad

122   Buckwheat Noodle Salad

123   Lentil Salad with Cucumber and Fennel

124   Asparagus and Shrimp Salad

125   Rice Salad

126   Rice, Lentil, and Olive Salad

127   Caesar Salad

128   Mung Bean Salad

129   Cauliflower and Broccoli Salad

130   My Favourite Herb Dressing

131   Sunflower Dressing

132   French Dressing

133   Simple Olive Oil Dressing

134   Italian Dressing

135   Thai Dressing

136   Basil and Red Pepper Dressing

137   Dairy-Free Caesar Dressing

138   Soyannaise

139   Creamy Cucumber Dressing

140   Pesto

141   Vegetable Stuffing

142   Beef Marinade

143   Chicken Marinade

144   Lamb Marinade

145   Chicken Salsa

Ingredients

1 cup	quinoa (250 ml)
2 cups	water (500 ml)
1/2 tsp	sea salt (2 ml)

Dressing:

1 tsp	sea salt (5 ml)
1/3-1/2 cup	olive oil (75-125 ml)
1/3 cup	lemon juice (75 ml)
2	cloves garlic, minced
1/2 cup	fresh mint, finely chopped (125 ml)
2 cups	fresh parsley, finely chopped (500 ml)
1	bunch green onions, finely chopped
1	carrot, diced
1	red pepper, diced, or 2 tomatoes, diced (optional)

Quinoa Salad

Free of dairy products, wheat, yeast, corn, sugar, eggs, soy, nuts, and gluten.

- Wash quinoa well and drain. In a pot, cover quinoa with 2 cups (500 ml) water and 1/2 tsp (2 ml) sea salt, bring to a boil, and simmer for 15-20 minutes. Once done, fluff cooked quinoa with a fork and set aside to let cool.

- Mix dressing ingredients together in a bowl and pour over the cooled quinoa; mix well and refrigerate.

Serve on a bed of lettuce with radicchio, or just on crackers or bread.

Yields 8 cups (2 L).

Sweet Potato Salad

Free of dairy products, wheat, yeast, corn, sugar, eggs, soy, nuts, nightshades, and gluten.

- Cook sweet potatoes until tender but not mushy. Cool potatoes, and put in bowl.
- Mix all ingredients together and enjoy.

Yields 4 1/2 cups (1.125 L).

Ingredients

4	sweet potatoes, peeled and cubed
2 Tbsp	olive oil or apple juice (30 ml)
3 Tbsp	lemon juice (45 ml)
1	clove garlic, minced
1 Tbsp	parsley, chopped (15 ml)
1 Tbsp	basil, chopped (15 ml)
1 Tbsp	chives, chopped (15 ml)
1	green onion, chopped

Potato Salad

Free of dairy products, wheat, yeast, corn, sugar, eggs, nuts, and gluten.

Ingredients

5	medium potatoes
1	large english cucumber, diced
	Soy mayonnaise
	Handful of fresh chives
	Sea salt to taste

- Slice potatoes in half and boil for 20 minutes or until slightly soft.

  Do not overcook potatoes, as you want to be able to slice them into cubes without crumbling.

- Dice cooked, cooled potatoes and place in a bowl. Add diced cucumber and cut-up chives and mix with your favourite mayonnaise.

  Refrigerate and serve cold.

  I invite you to use red potatoes in this recipe, as I find they have a lovely flavour.

Yields 5 cups (1.25 L).

Fruit Salad

Free of dairy products, wheat, yeast, corn, sugar, eggs, soy, nuts, nightshades, and gluten.

- With a melon baller (a great tool to have in your kitchen), ball out a cantaloupe, honeydew melon, and watermelon. Add any other fruits in season, such as strawberries, bananas, grapes, pineapple, peaches, blueberries, or nectarines.

- Let cut fruit sit in the refrigerator for at least 2 hours so that the juice comes out of the fruit.

  Serve cold.

Ingredients

1	cantaloupe
1	honeydew melon
1	watermelon
1	banana
	Other seasonal fruits

Good Ol. Fashioned Cabbage Salad

Free of dairy products, wheat, yeast, corn, sugar, eggs, nuts, nightshades, and gluten.

Ingredients

1/2	cabbage, grated or shredded
3-4	carrots, grated or shredded
	Soy mayonnaise or mayonnaise you can tolerate
	Sea salt to taste

- In a food processor, shred cabbage and carrots. You want the mixture to be half cabbage and half carrots.

  If you like, you can cut up a green pepper or a Vidalia onion as well, but I like just the carrots and cabbage on their own.

- Add your favourite mayonnaise, salt, and pepper to taste if you like, toss, and serve cold.

Yields 3 cups (750 ml).

Waldorf Salad

Free of dairy products, wheat, yeast, corn, sugar, eggs, and gluten.

- Cook and cool your rice first. Sometimes I cook my rice the night before, as it is easier and less time consuming.

- Wash and pull apart spinach leaves and put into a large bowl.

- Add all other ingredients and squeeze lemon juice over mixture.

- To make the dressing, mix tamari, olive oil, and garlic.

- Drizzle dressing over vegetable mixture.

- Cover and let marinate for 1 hour before serving.

Yields 10 cups (2.5 L) or 6-8 servings.

NOTE
You can substitute any grain you wish for the rice, such as cooked millet, kasha, or bulgur.

Ingredients

1 to 2	bunches of fresh spinach, cleaned and pulled apart into pieces
	Juice of 1/2 lemon
2 cups	cooked and cooled long grain brown rice (500 ml)
1/3 cup	raisins (75 ml)
1 cup	bean or lentil sprouts (250 ml)
3	stalks celery, chopped
1	red or green pepper, chopped
1/4 cup	fresh parsley, finely chopped (50 ml)
1/4 cup	green onions, chopped (50 ml)
1 cup	walnuts, cashews, or almonds (250 ml)

Dressing:

1/4 cup	wheat-free tamari (50 ml)
1/2 cup	olive oil (125 ml)
1-2	cloves garlic, minced

Buckwheat Noodle Salad

Free of dairy products, wheat, yeast, corn, sugar, eggs, soy, nuts, and gluten.

Ingredients

1	red pepper
	Package of buckwheat soba noodles, 250 grams (these are wheat-free noodles)
2 cups	broccoli, cut into bite-size pieces (500 ml)
	Lettuce leaves, enough for decoration

Herb Dressing:

3 Tbsp	olive oil (45 ml)
2 Tbsp	sesame oil (30 ml)
1 tsp	fresh ginger, grated (5 ml)
2	cloves garlic, minced
1 Tbsp	fresh parsley, chopped (15 ml)
1 Tbsp	each of basil, tarragon, chives, and thyme, chopped (15 ml)
	Sea salt and pepper to taste

- Cut and halve red pepper. Take seeds out. Roast red pepper on a barbeque grill or broil in oven until soft and skin is blackened.

- Place roasted pepper in paper bag, seal, and let sit for 10 minutes. If you do not have a paper bag, simply cover the cooked pepper with a linen towel, so the steam gets trapped in. This will make the skin come off easier. Scrape skin from pepper and cut into strips.

- In a large pot of boiling water, cook noodles until tender yet firm, about 10 minutes; drain and rinse under cold water.

- Blanch broccoli in boiling water for 2 minutes; drain and rinse under cold water.

- In a bowl, combine dressing ingredients and mix well. In larger bowl, combine cooled noodles and broccoli and strips of roasted red pepper, then mix in dressing.

  Serve on lettuce leaves.

Yields 4 cups.

NOTE
Look for buckwheat noodles in your local health food store, or Indian or Asian store.

Lentil Salad with Cucumber and Fennel

Free of dairy products, wheat, yeast, corn, sugar, eggs, soy, nuts, nightshades, and gluten.

- In a large pot, cover lentils with water, bring to boil, and then simmer for 20 minutes or until tender, then drain and set aside.

- In a skillet, cook green onions, carrot, fennel, and cumin in 2 tablespoons of water, cover, and simmer for 5 minutes. Set aside.

- In a salad bowl, combine lentils, carrot mixture, parsley, and cucumber. Drizzle olive oil and lemon juice over salad, add salt and pepper and mix.

Yields 5 cups.

DID YOU KNOW?
Fennel is often referred to as sweet anise, causing those who do not like the flavour of licorice to avoid it. The flavour of fennel is lighter than anise and when cooked is even sweeter.

Ingredients

1 cup	brown lentils (250 ml)
1/2 cup	green onions, sliced (125 ml)
1	carrot, sliced
1/4-1/2 cup	fennel, chopped (50-125 ml)
1 tsp	cumin (5 ml)
2 Tbsp	water (30 ml)
1/4 cup	fresh parsley, chopped (50 ml)
1 cup	cucumber, diced (250 ml)
2 Tbsp	white wine vinegar or lemon juice (30 ml)
1-2 tsp	olive oil (5-10 ml)
	Sea salt and pepper to taste

Asparagus and Shrimp Salad

Free of dairy products, wheat, yeast, corn, sugar, eggs, soy, nuts, nightshades, and gluten.

Ingredients

1	bunch asparagus
1	dozen shrimp, shelled and de-veined
8	lettuce leaves
5 Tbsp	olive oil (75 ml)
2 Tbsp	lemon juice (30 ml)
1 Tbsp	green onions, chopped finely (15 ml)
	Sea salt and pepper to taste

- Cook asparagus until tender. When done, rinse under cold water.

  This stops the cooking process. You can buy precooked shrimp, which will make this recipe a snap.

- You can also buy uncooked shrimp and simply throw shrimp in boiling water for a few minutes until they turn pink.

- Once shrimp are cooked, rinse in cold water. Arrange shrimp onto lettuce leaves and place asparagus on top of shrimp.

- Combine olive oil, lemon juice, green onions, salt, and pepper and whisk until the dressing thickens. Pour over shrimp and serve.

Yields 2 servings.

Rice Salad

Free of dairy products, wheat, yeast, corn, sugar, eggs, soy, nuts, and gluten.

- Mix all ingredients together and refrigerate.

  I like to use basmati rice in this recipe, as it has a lovely flavour. This makes a great summer salad.

Yields 4 cups (1 L).

Ingredients

3 cups	cooked rice (750 ml)
3/4 cup	cooked peas (175 ml)
1/4 cup	green pepper, diced (50 ml)
2 Tbsp	parsley, chopped (30 ml)
2 Tbsp	green onions or chives, chopped (30 ml)
	Fresh dill to taste

DID YOU KNOW?

That rice is thought to have been cultivated since at least 5000 B.C., and archeological explorations in China have uncovered sealed pots of rice that are over 8,000 years old.

Rice, Lentil and Olive Salad

Free of dairy products, wheat, yeast, corn, sugar, eggs, soy, nuts, nightshades, and gluten.

Ingredients

1 cup	basmati rice (250 ml)
2	cloves garlic, minced
1 cup	dried brown lentils (250 ml)
1/2	onion
2	bay leaves
1 cup	pimento-stuffed green olives, sliced (250 ml)
1/2 tsp	sea salt (2 ml)
1/4 tsp	pepper (1 ml)

Dressing:

3 Tbsp	olive oil (45 ml)
2 Tbsp	lemon juice (30 ml)
1 Tbsp	Dijon mustard or regular yellow mustard (15 ml)
1 tsp	dried thyme (5 ml)
	Pepper to taste
4	green onions, sliced

- To cook rice, bring 2 cups of water to a boil. Add rice, garlic, salt, and pepper, bring again to a boil, and cover. Reduce to a low heat and simmer for 20 minutes, until water is absorbed and rice is tender.

- Allow rice to stand in pot for 10 minutes, fluff with fork, then transfer to a bowl and let sit in refrigerator to cool a bit.

- Meanwhile, sort and wash lentils. Bring 4 cups water to a boil along with half of an onion and bay leaves, then add lentils.

- Return to a boil and then turn to low and simmer 20 minutes, until lentils are tender. Don't overcook, as the lentils will go mushy.

- Drain lentils and discard bay leaf and onion. Set lentils aside to cool. Whisk together the oil, lemon juice, mustard, thyme, pepper, and shallots.

- In a bowl combine cooled lentils, rice, dressing, and olives.

Refrigerate for several hours or overnight to allow the flavours to blend in. You could make this the day before and serve the following day.

Yields 5 cups.

Caesar Salad

Free of dairy products, wheat, yeast, corn, sugar, eggs, nuts, nightshades, and gluten.

- Clean and wash romaine lettuce.

- Shred lettuce into small pieces and put in salad bowl.

- Blend all dressing ingredients together in food processor until very smooth.

- Mix dressing into lettuce.

  If you can tolerate bread, make some croutons from your favourite bread to top your Caesar.
  This can also be used as a veggie dip as it is quite thick.

Yields 3 cups (750 ml).

Ingredients

1	head romaine lettuce
Dressing:	
1	block silken tofu
3 Tbsp	olive oil (45 ml)
2-3	garlic cloves, minced
1/2 cup	water (125 ml)
1/2 cup	watercress or parsley (125 ml)
1 tsp	dry mustard or turmeric (5 ml)
1 tsp	sea salt (5 ml)
	Juice from 2 lemons

DID YOU KNOW?
"Caesar Salad" is said to have been created in 1924 by Italian chef Caesar Cardini, who owned a restaurant in Tijuana, Mexico.

Mung Bean Salad

Free of dairy products, wheat, yeast, corn, sugar, eggs, nuts, and gluten.

Ingredients

1 cup	mung beans (250 ml)
1 cup	carrots, diced (250 ml)
1/2 cup	red pepper, diced (125 ml)
2	stalks celery, diced
1	english cucumber, diced
1 cup	fresh parsley, chopped (250 ml)

Dressing:

1	clove garlic, minced
1 Tbsp	fresh ginger, grated (15 ml)
1/4 cup	wheat-free tamari (50 ml)
1/8 cup	toasted sesame oil or sesame oil (25 ml)
	Half of 1 lemon, squeezed

- In a pot with 2 1/2 cups water, bring mung beans to a boil, simmer for 45-60 minutes or until mung beans are soft.

- Place cooked mung beans in a glass bowl and set aside to cool.

- Cut up vegetables and mix in with cooled mung beans.

- Mix dressing ingredients together and pour over mixture and cool for 1 hour before serving.

- This salad can be served warm or cold. In the winter I like to stir fry all vegetables except cucumber and mix in with warm mung beans, but in the summertime it is nice to have them all cool and crisp.

Yields 8 cups (2 L) or 6 servings.

NOTE

You can also make this with mung bean noodles. They are clear in colour and can be found in an Indian, Asian, or local health food store. Mung beans do not need to be pre-soaked.

Cauliflower and Broccoli Salad

Free of dairy products, wheat, yeast, corn, sugar, eggs, soy, nuts, and gluten.

- Cut up broccoli and cauliflower and blanch them (place in boiling water for about 3 minutes then remove and rinse under cold water; this will stop the cooking process right away).
- Mix all vegetables in a bowl and add olive oil, lemon juice, garlic, and umeboshi vinegar.

Yields 12 cups (3 L) or 6 servings.

NOTE

You can purchase umeboshi vinegar or paste in your local health food store. It is good for sauces and dressings and can be kept in your refrigerator for quite a long time.

DID YOU KNOW?

umeboshi plums grow in the northern regions of Japan. They have a somewhat sour and salty taste and are said to help calm stomach upset and detoxify the body.

Ingredients

1	head cauliflower, cut into flowerettes
1	head broccoli, cut into flowerettes
1	red pepper, diced
1	orange pepper, diced
1	yellow pepper, diced
3	carrots, sliced
	Handful fresh parsley, chopped
	Handful fresh basil, chopped
5 Tbsp	olive oil (75 ml)
2	cloves garlic, minced
3 Tbsp	umeboshi vinegar (45 ml)
	Juice of 1 lemon
	Sea salt to taste

My Favourite Herb Dressing

Free of dairy products, wheat, yeast, corn, sugar, eggs, soy, nuts, nightshades, and gluten.

Ingredients

2	cloves garlic, minced
1 tsp	dry mustard (5 ml)
1/2 cup	red wine vinegar (125 ml)
4	strips anchovies, or 1 tsp anchovy paste
1 cup	olive oil (250 ml)
2 Tbsp	fresh parsley, chopped (30 ml)
	Dash oregano
	Dash basil
	Dash sea salt
	Dash pepper

- Mix all ingredients together in a blender or food processor, refrigerate, and serve.

Yields 1 1/2 cups (375 ml).

NOTE Salad Dressings are great to have on hand. Keep a few glass jars around, as Dressings keep well in them.

DID YOU KNOW?
Anchovies once opened can be stored in oil in an airtight container in the refrigerator for up to 2 months. To reduce their saltiness, soak in cool water for 30 minutes.

Sunflower Dressing

Free of dairy products, wheat, yeast, corn, sugar, eggs, soy, nuts, and gluten.

Ingredients

1 cup	roasted sunflower seeds (250 ml)
1	clove garlic, minced
1/2	red pepper, roasted
1/2 tsp	sea salt (2 ml)
3/4 cup	water (175 ml)
	Juice of 1/2 lemon

- Roast raw sunflower seeds in cast-iron pan on low to medium heat until nicely browned. Stir frequently so they don't burn.

- Roast red pepper in oven, under broiler, until skins blacken; cool, then peel off skin.

- Blend all ingredients together in food processor, adding water slowly — you don't want it too runny.

  This is a great dressing for potatoes or for avocados, or for a dip with raw veggies.

Yields 2 cups (500 ml).

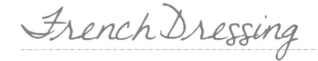

French Dressing

Free of dairy products, wheat, yeast, corn, sugar, eggs, soy, nuts, nightshades, and gluten.

Ingredients

1/2 cup	olive oil (125 ml)
	Juice of 1 lemon
4 Tbsp	apple cider vinegar (60 ml)
1	clove garlic, minced
	Dash salt and pepper
2 Tbsp	parsley (30 ml)
2 Tbsp	chives (30 ml)
2 Tbsp	basil (30 ml)
1 Tbsp	honey (15 ml)

- Blend ingredients well, or shake in glass jar.

  In the summer it is lovely to use fresh parsley, chives, and basil. Just make sure you cut them very fine for this recipe.

Yields 1 cup (250 ml).

Simple Olive Oil Dressing

Free of dairy products, wheat, yeast, corn, sugar, eggs, soy, nuts, nightshades, and gluten.

Ingredients

3 Tbsp	lemon juice (45 ml)
1 Tbsp	dry mustard (15 ml)
2	cloves garlic, minced
1/2 cup	olive oil or canola oil (125 ml)
	Add any herbs you can tolerate (basil, mint, ginger)
	Salt and pepper

- Mix lemon juice with mustard and garlic.

- Slowly add oil while stirring until oil is blended.

- Then add whichever herbs you wish, salt and pepper if you like, and serve.

Yields 1 cup (250 ml).

Ingredients

2	cloves garlic, minced
1 tsp	dried tarragon (5 ml)
1 tsp	dried marjoram (5 ml)
1 tsp	dry mustard (5 ml)
1/2 cup	olive oil, canola or vegetable oil (125 ml)
1 Tbsp	red wine vinegar (15 ml)
1/2 tsp	sea salt (2 ml)
1/4 tsp	pepper (1 ml)

Italian Dressing

Free of dairy products, wheat, yeast, corn, sugar, eggs, soy, nuts, nightshades, and gluten.

- Combine all ingredients in glass jar with tight lid and shake well.

- Let stand at room temperature for 1 hour and then refrigerate.

- Shake well before serving.

  This is a great dressing for potatoes, rice, pasta, or a mixed salad.

Yields 1/2 cup (125 ml).

Thai Dressing

Free of dairy products, wheat, yeast, corn, sugar, eggs, soy, nuts, nightshades, and gluten.

- Mix all ingredients together in a food processor and keep refrigerated in a dark container until you are ready to use.

- Pour over lentils or use as a vinaigrette sauce for cold potato salad, rice, or lentils.

Yields 1/2 cup (125 ml).

Ingredients

1/2 cup	sesame oil (125 ml)
	Dash roasted sesame oil
2 Tbsp	fresh mint, chopped (30 ml)
2 Tbsp	fresh coriander, chopped (30 ml)
4 tsp	fresh ginger, grated (20 ml)
3	green onions, chopped
1/2 tsp	cumin or curry powder (2 ml)
	Sea salt and pepper to taste

Basil and Red Pepper Dressing

Free of dairy products, wheat, yeast, corn, sugar, eggs, soy, nuts, and gluten.

Ingredients

1	bunch basil, finely cut
1	large red pepper, cut into fine strips
1/2 cup	rice wine vinegar (125 ml)
1/2 cup	flaxseed oil (125 ml)
1/2 cup	sunflower oil (125 ml)
	Juice of 1 lemon
1	clove garlic, minced
	Sea salt to taste

- Mix all ingredients in the blender or your food processor and serve.

Yields 2 1/2 cups (625 ml).

DID YOU KNOW?

That basil was once called the "royal herb" by the Greeks. To store basil, wrap in damp paper towels in a plastic bag and refrigerate for up to 4 days.

Dairy-Free Caesar Dressing

Free of dairy products, wheat, yeast, corn, sugar, eggs, nuts, nightshades, and gluten.

- Mix all ingredients in a blender or whip in a bowl with a whisk.
- Store in a dark bottle in the fridge.

Yields 1 cup (250 ml).

Ingredients

1/2 cup	olive oil (125 ml)
1/2 cup	flaxseed oil (125 ml)
3 Tbsp	lemon juice (45 ml)
3	cloves garlic, minced
1 tsp	yellow mustard (5 ml)
1 tsp	wheat-free tamari (5 ml)
2	anchovies
2 Tbsp	ground sunflower seeds (30 ml)
1/4 tsp	sea salt (1 ml)

Ingredients

1 cup	silken tofu (250 ml)
1/2 cup	oil (your choice) (125 ml)
2 Tbsp	onion, finely chopped (30 ml)
3 Tbsp	lemon juice (45 ml)
1/2 tsp	paprika (2 ml)
1/4 tsp	dry mustard or cayenne (1 ml)
1 tsp	honey (5 ml)
1/4 tsp	salt (1 ml)

Soyannaise

Free of dairy products, wheat, yeast, corn, sugar, eggs, nuts, nightshades, and gluten. Paprika and cayenne are part of the nightshade family, so omit if necessary.

- Mix all ingredients in blender except oil and lemon juice. Add oil very slowly while blending; add lemon juice and blend again.

- Refrigerate and serve.

  Great spread for toast with a sliced avocado, or on a tomato sandwich.

Yields 1 cup (250 ml).

Creamy Cucumber Dressing

Free of dairy products, wheat, yeast, corn, sugar, eggs, nightshades, and gluten.

Ingredients

1 cup	silken or smooth tofu (250 ml)
1/4 cup	lime juice (50 ml)
1	cucumber, sliced
1/4 cup	cashews (50 ml)
2	green onions, chopped
3 Tbsp	fresh dill (45ml)
1/2 tsp	sea salt (2 ml)

- In a food processor, grind cashews until very fine, add all other ingredients and blend until dressing is smooth and creamy.

- Refrigerate and serve.

  This makes quite a thick dressing. I also use it as a dip for veggies. For a smoother consistency, use silken tofu.

Yields 3 cups (750 ml).

Pesto

Free of dairy products, wheat, yeast, corn, sugar, eggs, soy, nightshades, and gluten.

Ingredients

1/4 cup	pine nuts (50 ml)
1	bunch fresh basil
1/2	bunch fresh parsley
1	bunch fresh spinach
1/4 cup	olive oil (50 ml)
2-3	cloves garlic, crushed
1/2 tsp	sea salt (2 ml)
1-2 Tbsp	lemon juice (15-30 ml)

I love this in the summertime when the basil, spinach, and parsley are fresh. It is relatively easy to make in your food processor and then you have it on hand and can either freeze it or keep it in the fridge for a few days. Simply boil your favourite wheat-free pasta and mix in pesto.

- Roast pine nuts in cast-iron frying pan. No oil is necessary. Be patient and cook on low heat, stirring pine nuts so they don't burn. Pine nuts are done when they turn a golden colour.

- Clean and rinse well, basil, parsley, and spinach and remove stems. Dry well between paper towels or clean tea towel.

- In a food processor, mix basil, parsley, spinach, olive oil, garlic, sea salt, lemon juice, and a few of the roasted pine nuts.

- Your mixture should have a thick, pasty consistency. If you find it too dry, add a little water or a bit more lemon juice or oil.

- Add pesto to your favourite pasta. Top pasta and pesto with remaining roasted pine nuts.

Yields 2 cups (500 ml).

Vegetable Stuffing

Free of dairy products, wheat, yeast, corn, sugar, eggs, soy, nuts, and nightshades. If you use yeast-free bread, this a yeast-free recipe.

- In a large skillet, sauté onion in oil for a few minutes. Add mushrooms and celery.

- Cook over medium heat until mushrooms begin to brown, then add the bread and seasonings.

- Lower heat and continue to cook for 5 minutes. Stir in stock a little at a time until dressing obtains desired moistness.

- Place in a lightly oiled 9x13-inch baking dish, cover, and bake for 20 minutes at 350F.

- Remove lid and bake for another 10 minutes.

Yields 4 cups (1 L).

Ingredients

1	medium onion, finely chopped
3 Tbsp	olive oil (45 ml)
3 cups	mushrooms, sliced (750 ml)
1 cup	celery, sliced (250 ml)
4 cups	bread crumbs (wheat-free bread) (1 L)
1 cup	vegetable stock (250 ml)
1/4 cup	fresh parsley, chopped (50 ml)
1/4 tsp	sage (1 ml)
1/4 tsp	thyme (1 ml)
1/8 tsp	marjoram (.5 ml)
1/8 tsp	black pepper (.5 ml)
1/2 tsp	sea salt (2 ml)

Ingredients

2/3 cup	lemon juice (150 ml)
1/3 cup	canola oil (75 ml)
4	cloves garlic, minced
2 tsp	oregano (10 ml)
1/2	medium onion, sliced
	Pepper to taste

Beef Marinade

Free of dairy products, wheat, yeast, corn, sugar, eggs, soy, nuts, nightshades, and gluten.

- Mix ingredients together and blend with hand-held blender so that flavours mix and become liquidy.

- Marinate large chunks of sirloin steak, about 2 pounds for this recipe.

- Let sit in marinade for at least 4 hours in the refrigerator.

- Skewer meat with cut-up vegetables and barbeque on grill.

  I tend to use zucchini, red pepper, and onions for my skewers.

Yields 1 1/2 cups (375 ml), enough marinade for 2-3 pounds sirloin.

Chicken Marinade

Free of dairy products, wheat, yeast, corn, sugar, eggs, nuts, nightshades, and gluten.

Ingredients

1 cup	organic apple juice (250 ml)
1/2 cup	tamari (wheat-free soy sauce) (125 ml)
1 Tbsp	honey (15 ml)
2 Tbsp	olive oil (30 ml)
1	clove garlic, minced

- Mix all ingredients together and use as a marinade for chicken.

Yields 2 cups (500 ml).

Lamb Marinade

Free of dairy products, wheat, yeast, corn, sugar, eggs, nuts, nightshades, and gluten.

Ingredients

1/2 cup	lemon juice (125 ml)
2 Tbsp	dry mustard (mixed in a bit of water) (30 ml)
1 cup	vegetable stock (250 ml)
1/2 cup	tamari (wheat-free soy sauce) (125 ml)
2	cloves garlic, minced
2 Tbsp	horseradish (30 ml)
	Pepper to taste

- Mix all ingredients together. Place lamb in a glass pan with marinade and let marinate for at least 3 hours in the fridge. Barbeque or roast lamb in the oven.

Yields 2 cups (500 ml) and will be enough to marinate 4-6 shoulder chops or a small lamb roast.

NOTE

You can use this on a lamb roast or lamb shoulder chops. I try to buy fresh horseradish and grate it myself, as I find that most of the store-bought horseradishes have too many extras in them that I cannot tolerate.

Chicken Salsa

Free of dairy products, wheat, yeast, corn, sugar, eggs, soy, nuts, nightshades, and gluten.

- In a blender, blend mango and peach, add lime juice, salt, and pepper and spread over cooked chicken breast.

Yields 2 cups (500 ml).

Ingredients

2	peaches, sliced
1	mango, sliced
	Juice of 1 lime
1 tsp	honey (5 ml)
	Sea salt and pepper to taste

Snacks
and Spreads

148   Yummy Red Lentil Dip

149   Sesame Crackers

150   Crispies

151   Good Ol' Hummus

152   Sweet Potato Pâté

154   Vegetarian Pâté

155   Carrot Loaf

156   Nibble Mix

157   Homemade Fries

158   Garbanzo Spread

159   Parsnip Spread

160   Eggplant Dip or Pasta Sauce

161   Tofu Spread

162   White Bean Dip

163   Pizza

Yummy Red Lentil Dip

Free of dairy products, wheat, yeast, corn, sugar, eggs, soy, nuts, nightshades, and gluten.

Ingredients

1 cup	organic red lentils (250 ml)
1	medium organic onion, chopped
2	bay leaves
2-3	cloves garlic, minced
1/2	lemon, sqeezed
1 1/2 tsp	dried tarragon (7 ml)
1/2 tsp	sea salt (2 ml)
3 cups	water (750 ml)
	Pepper to taste

This is a simple, nutritious dip and very easy to make in your food processor.

- Wash red lentils and remove any foreign objects. Sometimes you will find little stones in with the lentils.

- Bring 3 cups (750 ml) water to a boil and add the red lentils, chopped onions, and bay leaves. Bring to a boil and then reduce heat and simmer for 20 minutes or until tender. Drain lentils through a sieve and discard bay leaves.

- Put lentils in blender or food processor. Add garlic, lemon juice, olive oil, tarragon, salt, and pepper. Puree until smooth.

- Pour into serving dish and refrigerate.

Serve with cut-up vegetables, rice crackers, or chips . . . A great dip!

Yields 3 cups (750 ml).

Sesame Crackers

Free of dairy products, wheat, yeast, corn, sugar, eggs, soy, nuts, and nightshades.

Ingredients

1/2 cup	warm water (125 ml)
1/3 cup	sunflower or safflower oil (75 ml)
1/2-1 tsp	herbal salt or sea salt (2-5 ml)
1 3/4 cup	oat flour (425 ml)
1/4 cup	oat bran (50 m)
1/2 cup	sesame seeds (125 ml)
1 Tbsp	flax seeds (15 ml)

I buy herbal salt at my local health food store. It is simply sea salt with dried herbs in it.

Besides rice crackers, I have not been able to find any store-bought crackers that I can eat, as they all contain ingredients that I am allergic to; so these are a nice change.

- In a food processor, mix water, oil, and salt. Add oat flour, oat bran, and sesame seeds and mix.

- Then place mixture in a bowl and with your hands knead a little and then let sit in the bowl for 20 minutes. I usually cover it with a tea towel and try to find a warm place for it. You can always turn on your oven to 150F and then turn it off and place the bowl in the oven for the 20 minutes.

- Flatten onto baking sheet, I use pizza pan or a small cookie sheet.

- Sprinkle with a bit more herbal salt and cook for 20-25 minutes at 350F. Remove and let cool and then break into pieces.

- Use crackers with any of the dips or spreads found in this cookbook or simply mash some avocadoes and top with that.

Yields 1 small cookie sheet or pizza pan.

NOTE
I make this recipe with Kamut as well. Simply substitute Kamut flour for oat flour and Kamut flakes for oat bran. Make sure you grind your Kamut flakes to the consistency of bran.

Crispies

Free of dairy products, wheat, yeast, corn, sugar, eggs, soy, nightshades, and gluten.

Ingredients

2 cups	brown rice, crispy cereal, or puffed rice (500 ml)
1/2 cup	brown rice syrup or barley malt (125 ml)
1/3 cup	raisins (75 ml)
1/2 cup	crunchy peanut butter (50ml)
1/3 cup	sunflower seeds (75 ml)
1/4 cup	pepitas (pumpkin seeds) (50 ml)

Brown rice crispy cereal is the healthy option to Rice Krispies™, as it has no added sugar or additives. You can purchase it at your local health food store.

- Place rice syrup and peanut butter in a saucepan and heat; do not boil. If you are using peanuts instead of peanut butter, just heat syrup alone.

- Place all other ingredients in a bowl. Pour hot rice syrup over the ingredients and mix in.

- Line an 8x8-inch square pan with waxed paper. Place mixture in pan and with wet hands or spatula pat down and flatten. Put in fridge to harden for 30 minutes before eating.

- Slice into squares and enjoy.

Yields 1 pan.

NOTE

You can add any seeds to this snack, such as sesame seeds or flax seeds. You can also use puffed rice, puffed millet, or puffed quinoa as alternatives. If you want this to be gluten free, use rice syrup, not barley malt.

Good Ol' Hummus

Free of dairy products, wheat, yeast, corn, sugar, eggs, soy, nuts, nightshades, and gluten. If you use the roasted red pepper, then you will have nightshades in this recipe.

Ingredients

1 can	cooked chickpeas or garbanzo beans (14 fl.oz can, 398 ml)
1	clove garlic, minced
	Juice of 1 lemon
2 Tbsp	tahini (30 ml)
3-5 Tbsp	olive oil (45-75 ml)
1 tsp	cumin (5ml)
1	whole roasted red pepper (optional)

- To roast pepper, cut red pepper in half, clean out insides, place face down on tray, and broil in oven on top rack until skins have blackened. Place in paper bag until cool and peel off black skin. If you do not have a paper bag, simply place a tea towel over the grilled pepper for a few minutes. This will trap the steam so the skin peels off easily.

- Blend all ingredients together in a food processor until smooth. If mixture is too thick, add some more olive oil or lemon juice. With this recipe, I do not cook my chickpeas from scratch. I cheat and buy canned organic garbanzo beans from my local health food store.

- If you are cooking your beans from scratch, see note on page 44.

  You know, I never liked hummus, but now that I add roasted red pepper to it, it gives it a lovely flavour and I love it. Try it with rice crackers or sliced, raw veggies.

Yields 2 cups (500 ml).

Sweet Potato Pâté

Free of dairy products, wheat, yeast, corn, sugar, eggs, soy, nuts, and gluten. If you want this recipe to be free of nightshades, use all sweet potatoes.

Ingredients

2 cups	roasted raw sunflower seeds (500 ml)
1	sweet potato
1	white potato
1	onion, chopped fine and sautéed in olive oil with garlic
2-3	cloves garlic, minced
1 tsp	sea salt (5 ml)
1 tsp	savory (5 ml)
1 tsp	thyme (5 ml)
3 Tbsp	olive oil (optional) (45 ml)
1	carrot, peeled
1	celery stalk, diced
2 cups	water (500 ml)

- Cut up and cook potatoes in about 2 cups of water. When done, save the cooking water.

- Roast sunflower seeds by toasting them over a low to medium heat in a cast-iron pan, until golden. Do not add anything. Stir continuously so they do not burn.

- In your food processor, blend the roasted sunflower seeds until they are very fine.

- After you have roasted your sunflower seeds in your cast-iron pan, simply wipe out pan and sauté onion in olive oil, with minced garlic, savory, and thyme. You can throw in some grated carrot, diced celery, or zucchini if you wish at the last minute. You want the carrot, celery, and zucchini to be crunchy, so don't cook too long.

- Mash potatoes using leftover cooking water, or oil if using any. Add ground sunflower seeds, salt, cooked onions, and veggies. If the mixture is dry, add a bit of potato water that you saved.

- Mix well and put in loaf pan to cook at 350 F for about one hour or until golden.

Sweet Potato Pâté

- Let cool and refrigerate. Remove and slice.

  Delicious on rice crackers, veggies, or toast, or serve with a salad.

- Wrap pieces in plastic wrap and freeze if keeping more than 3 days.

Yields 1 loaf.

Vegetarian Pâté

Free of dairy products, wheat, yeast, corn, sugar, eggs, soy, and nuts. You can make this recipe gluten free if you use rice flour instead of spelt.

Ingredients

1 cup	hulled raw organic sunflower seeds (250 ml)
1/2 cup	spelt flour (125 ml)
1	large onion, diced
1/4 cup	sunflower or safflower oil (50 ml)
2 Tbsp	lemon juice (30 ml)
1	medium potato, diced
1/2-1 cup	hot water (125-250 ml)
2 tsp	sea salt (10 ml)
1/2 tsp	thyme (2 ml)
2 tsp	basil (10 ml)
1/2 tsp	black pepper (2 ml)
1/2 tsp	sage (2 ml)

- In a food processor, grind sunflower seeds until they are relatively fine. Add flour, oil, lemon, some of the hot water, onion, potato, and herbs. Add water slowly, as you do not want to make mixture too watery and you may not need all of the water. Mix well and spoon into loaf pan.

  This is a great pâté to make to put on top of any type of crackers; or simply slice and serve with a salad for lunches when you have run out of lunch ideas.

- Bake at 350F for 1 hour in bread loaf pan.

  Let cool and serve.

Yields 1 loaf.

Carrot Loaf

Free of dairy products, wheat, yeast, corn, sugar, soy, and gluten.

- Grind nuts fairly fine and add all ingredients together and mix well.

- Put in a loaf pan and bake at 350F for approximately 30 minutes, until firm.

  Let cool and slice and serve with tossed salad or steamed vegetables.

Yields 1 loaf.

NOTE

I tend to use leftover rice in this recipe. If I am cooking rice the night before, I simply cook an extra cup of it and then have it on hand for this recipe or some of the others in this cookbook. I like to use roasted, unsalted cashews instead of raw cashews.

Ingredients

1 1/2 cup	cooked brown rice (375 ml)
1 1/2 cup	cashews or walnuts, ground (375 ml)
2 cups	carrots, grated (500 ml)
1	medium onion, finely chopped
1/4 cup	green pepper, finely chopped (50 ml)
1/4 cup	celery, finely chopped (50 ml)
2 tsp	fresh ground ginger (10 ml)
2 tsp	lemon juice (10 ml)
2 Tbsp	parsley, finely chopped (30 ml)
1	egg or egg substitute (use flaxseed or see substitute page)
	(2 Tbsp [30 ml] ground flaxseed to 6 Tbsp [90 ml] water)

Ingredients

Nuts

Seeds

Nibble Mix

Free of dairy products, wheat, yeast, corn, sugar, eggs, soy, nightshades, and gluten.

A nibble mix can be anything from homeroasted nuts and/or seeds such as almonds, hazelnuts, cashews, pecans, sunflower seeds, and pumpkin seeds.

If you roast them yourself, simply roast in a cast-iron frying pan. No need to add any oil. Stir frequently until nuts or seeds are golden.

You can also roast your nuts in the oven at 350F for 10 minutes, stir, then roast for another 5 minutes. Let cool and you can keep them in a glass jar in the fridge for at least a week.

If you don't want to roast your nuts, simply buy raw nuts or seeds at your local health food store and eat them when hunger attacks.

Great for afternoon snacks instead of a chocolate bar.

Homemade Fries

Free of dairy products, wheat, yeast, corn, sugar, eggs, soy, nuts, and gluten.

- Wash, peel, and cut potatoes into thick match-sticks. I usually count 2 large potatoes per person.

- Rinse cut potatoes in cold water and then dry potatoes well.

- Place on well-oiled cookie sheet and drizzle a bit of oil over them, so that they will not stick while cooking. You can also put potato strips in a bag with a little oil and shake it up. This will use less oil if you are watching your fat content.

- Cook in 400F oven for 30-40 minutes, turning them with a spatula often so they don't stick.

- When done, sprinkle with sea salt and lemon juice. Yummy!

  You can use sweet potatoes for this as well. They make great fries.

Ingredients

Potatoes

Olive oil

Sea salt

Garbanzo Spread

Free of dairy products, wheat, yeast, corn, sugar, eggs, soy, nuts, nightshades, and gluten.

Ingredients

1 can	garbanzo beans, drained (398ml)
2	green onions, chopped
1	clove garlic, minced
2 Tbsp	lemon juice (30 ml)
1/2 cup	olive oil (125 ml)
1/2 cup	parsley, chopped (125 ml)
1/2 tsp	dried (2 ml) or 1 Tbsp (15 ml) fresh basil
1/4 cup	sesame seeds (50 ml)

- Purée all ingredients in blender or food processor at low speed. If mixture is too thick, add a little water.

  Chill and serve with veggies.

Yields 2 cups (500 ml).

NOTE

Wash parsley well, as fresh parsley can sometimes be full of dirt. Pat dry and place parsley in a bowl. With scissors, cut parsley until very fine or cut in food processor.

Parsnip Spread

Free of dairy products, wheat, yeast, corn, sugar, eggs, nightshades, and gluten.

- Cook parsnips in a small amount of water until tender. Drain parsnips but retain some of the water. Mash parsnips with some of the leftover cooking water.

- Grind cashews in blender or food processor until very fine. Add in remaining ingredients and mix well, until smooth.

- Spoon into pâté dish.

  Garnish with parsley and serve with crackers or veggies.

Yields 3 cups (750 ml).

Ingredients

1 cup	parsnips, washed and sliced (250 ml)
1/2 cup	raw cashews (125 ml)
1 cup	cooked millet (250 ml)
1/2 cup	mashed tofu (125 ml)
1/2 cup	onion, finely chopped (125 ml)
1 tsp	basil (5 ml)
2 Tbsp	fresh parsley, chopped (30 ml)
1/2 cup	celery, chopped (125 ml)
2 Tbsp	water (from cooking the parsnips) (30 ml)
1 1/2 Tbsp	wheat-free tamari (22 ml)
1 Tbsp	olive oil (15 ml)
1/4 tsp	sea salt (1 ml)
1	pear (optional)

Eggplant Dip or Pasta Sauce

Free of dairy products, wheat, yeast, corn, sugar, eggs, soy, nuts, and gluten.

Ingredients

1	small red onion, diced
2	cloves garlic, minced
1	medium eggplant, chopped
1/2 cup	water (125 ml)
1/4 cup	olive oil (50 ml)
1/4 cup	lemon juice (50 ml)
2 Tbsp	fresh basil, minced, or 1 Tbsp dried basil (30 ml)
2 Tbsp	sesame seeds (30 ml)

- Sauté onion and garlic in a little olive oil. Add chopped eggplant, water, and a bit more oil.

- Cover and simmer for 10 minutes.

- Stir in remaining ingredients and then purée in food processor and chill.

Yields 3 cups (750 ml).

I think eggplants are sexy-looking. I don't know whether it is their colour, their shape, or perhaps their European name of Aubergine. Every Autumn, I go to the market and look at the lovely eggplants, onions, and fresh basil and think, now what can I make with eggplants? Well, here it is. This recipe makes a great dip for crackers and raw veggies, or simply add a little bit more water so its consistency is more like a sauce and use it over your favourite pasta. I love this over wheat-free kamut or rice pasta.

Tofu Spread

Free of dairy products, wheat, yeast, corn, sugar, eggs, nuts, nightshades, and gluten.

- Place all ingredients in food processor and blend until smooth. Add water or more olive oil if mixture is too dry.

- Cover and refrigerate.

  This spread will keep in the fridge for a few days. Use as a dip with raw vegetables or spread it on rice crackers or bread. A great substitute for cream cheese.

Yields 3 cups (750 ml).

Ingredients

1	block firm tofu
1/4 cup	fresh lemon juice (50 ml)
3-4 Tbsp	fresh dill (45-50 ml)
1/2 tsp	onion powder (optional) (2 ml)
1-2	cloves garlic, minced
2-3 Tbsp	fresh basil (30-45 ml)
2 Tbsp	hot water (30 ml)
1-2 Tbsp	olive oil (15-30 ml)
	Sea salt to taste

one of my taste testers had this to say about this dip.

"Dill Pseudo-cream cheese: Mmmmm! That's another winner. Plenty o' Dill. A virtual Dill fest. A Dill-o-rama! So, what the heck Did you say it was that I was eating?"

NOTE

They say that soy is very good for you and a good source of protein. This is an easy dip to make, and with fresh dill and basil, it has a lovely flavour and makes for a great substitute for cream cheese for those of us who have to avoid dairy.

White Bean Dip

Free of dairy products, wheat, yeast, corn, sugar, eggs, soy, nuts, nightshades, and gluten. Omit paprika if you wish to have this recipe free of nightshades.

Ingredients

1 can	lima beans, 14 fl oz. (398 ml)
1 Tbsp	dry mustard (15 ml)
1	small clove garlic, minced
2 Tbsp	fresh lemon juice (30 ml)
1/4 cup	olive oil or flaxseed oil (50 ml)
3 Tbsp	fresh parsley, chopped (45 ml)
	Paprika (optional)
	Sea salt to taste

Some of you may not care for lima beans, but try this recipe. I have never really liked lima beans on their own, but I love this dip.

- Place beans in a food processor with mustard, garlic, lemon juice, olive oil, parsley, and salt. Blend well and then spoon into a bowl.

If you use flaxseed oil, use the dip within a day or so. If you use olive oil, this can keep in the fridge for a few days. Sprinkle a dash of paprika on top if desired.

Serve with raw veggies or rice crackers.

Yields 2 cups (500 ml).

NOTE
My friend says this dip is addictive!

Pizza

Free of dairy products, wheat, yeast, corn, sugar, eggs, soy, nuts, and gluten.

Base:

- Mix dry ingredients together.
- Add water and mix with a fork.
- Press into a lightly greased pizza pan.

Topping:

- Spread tomato sauce over base.
- Sauté onions in oil until brown. Add onions, sliced red pepper and zucchini on top of tomato sauce. Bake at 350F for 30-40 minutes. You can also add in mushrooms, olives, or your choice of vegetables.

Yields 1 pizza.

Ingredients

Base:

3/4 cup	buckwheat flour (175 ml)
3/4 cup	brown rice flour (175 ml)
1/2 tsp	baking soda (2 ml)
1 tsp	cream of tartar (5 ml)
1/2-3/4 cup	water (125-175 ml)

Topping:

	Pasta Sauce
1	onion, sliced
1	red pepper, sliced
1	zucchini, sliced

NOTE
I buy organic tomato basil pasta sauce in a jar from my local health food store to use as a topping.

Desserts

166   Mum's Homemade Applesauce

167   Apple Pudding

168   Blueberry Muffins

169   Banana Muffins

170   Blueberry Banana Muffins

171   Apple Walnut Muffins

172   Peanut Butter Banana Muffins

173   Sweet Potato Dessert

174   Lemon Almond Biscotti

176   Banana Date Cookies

177   Fruit and Nut Bars

178   Gingerbread Cookies

179   Birthday Cake

180   Pseudo-Brownies

181   Pseudo-Brownie Icing

182   Date and Carob Icing

183   Carob Tahini Icing

184   Carrot Date Muffins

185   Cranberry Loaf

186   Sweet Potato Muffins

187   Fruit Mousse

188   Carob Banana Pie

189   Sunflower Oat Bars

190   Apple Crisp

191   Strawberry Hemp Ice

192   Carob Banana Hemp Ice

193   Oatmeal Cookies

194   Lime Coconut Cookies

195   Christmas Treats

196   Christmas Cashew Balls

197   Orange Teff Cookies

198   Teff Peanut Butter Cookies

199   Rice Pudding with Lemon

200   Barley Pudding

201   Carrot Haystacks

202   Carob Haystacks

203   Cashew Muffins

Mum's Homemade Applesauce

Free of dairy products, wheat, yeast, corn, sugar, eggs, soy, nuts, nightshades, and gluten.

Ingredients

12	organic apples
	Water

- Wash, core, and cut apples into small pieces. Leave skins on if apples are organic. Put enough water in bottom of pot so the apples do not burn. Bring to boil and let apples simmer until soft.

  Leaving the skins on will give applesauce a lovely pink colour if you are using red apples.

- When the apples are cooked, place through a strainer or just blend in blender or with hand blender so apple skins are puréed. You can add a dash of cinnamon if you like, or maple syrup, but I like it just plain.

  I used to love to watch my mum make applesauce when I was little. As she was cutting the apples, she would always give me a small piece of apple. Then the house would fill with the smell of cooked apples.

  There is nothing like a warm bowl of applesauce with a wheat-free cookie. Yum!

Yields 4 cups (1 L).

Apple Pudding

Free of dairy products, wheat, yeast, corn, sugar, eggs, soy, nuts, nightshades and gluten.

Ingredients

3	organic apples
1/4 cup	gluten-free rolled oats (50ml)
3/4 cup	organic apple juice (175 ml)
1/2 cup	water (125 ml)
1/2 cup	brown rice, cooked (125 ml)
1/4 tsp	cinnamon (1 ml)
1 Tbsp	rice syrup or maple syrup (15 ml)
	Dash nutmeg

- Core and slice your apples.

- Mix all ingredients in a saucepan and bring to boil, cover, and simmer for 20 minutes.

- Once apples are done, blend smoothly in a blender or food processor with another dash of cinnamon and nutmeg.

  You want it to be a nice smooth consistency, like that of a pudding.

  Serve topped with roasted nuts or seeds.

Yields 4 cups (1 L).

NOTE

This is a dessert that you will want to make just in time for dinner, as I find that once you put it in the fridge it becomes a bit clumpy due to the rice. You will have to reheat it on the stove or in your microwave if you make it the day before.

DID YOU KNOW?

That there are over a thousand varieties of apples and range in colour from yellow to green to crimson red.

Kamut or barley flakes work well in this recipe if you cannot have oats.

Wheat-Free Blueberry Muffins

Free of dairy products, wheat, yeast, corn, sugar, eggs, soy, nuts, and nightshades.

Ingredients

2 cups	spelt flour (or use 1 cup spelt with 3/4 cup brown rice flour) (500 ml)
2 tsp	baking powder (10 ml)
1-2 Tbsp	maple syrup, or honey, (15-30 ml) or substitute with 1/4 tsp (1 ml) Stevia
1 tsp	poppy seeds (5 ml)
	Pinch sea salt
1 cup	rice milk or soy milk (250 ml)
4 Tbsp	coconut oil or butter, melted (60 ml)
1	egg or egg replacer. I use flaxseed. (1 Tbsp [15 ml] flaxseed with 3/4 [175 ml] water. Bring to a boil. Let cool. Will get egg-like.)
	Rind of 1 organic lemon, or more to taste
	Juice of 1 lemon
1 cup	fresh or frozen organic blueberries, thawed and drained (250 ml)

- Preheat oven to 375 F.

- Lightly oil muffin pan.

- Combine flour, baking powder, poppy seeds, and salt in a large bowl and stir. Add rice milk, coconut oil, egg replacer, sweetener, lemon zest, and lemon juice and stir until moistened. Fold in blueberries.

- Spoon batter into muffin tins, filling two-thirds full. Bake for 20-25 minutes or until golden brown.

These muffins are great all year round, as you can buy frozen blueberries at any time at the grocery store. They are especially nice in the summer when you can get your blueberries fresh from the market.

Yields 12 muffins.

NOTE
See substitutes at the front of the book regarding Stevia and its use. Spelt and Kamut flour work in this recipe.

Banana Muffins

Free of dairy products, wheat, yeast, corn, sugar, eggs, soy, nuts, and nightshades.

Ingredients

2 cups	spelt flour (500 ml)
2 tsp	baking soda (10 ml)
1/2 tsp	vitamin C crystals (2 ml)
1/4 tsp	guar gum (1 ml)
1 1/2 tsp	cinnamon (7 ml)
4	large ripe mashed bananas with
1/4-1/2 cup	water (50-125 ml)
1/4 cup	safflower oil (50 ml)
1 Tbsp	maple syrup (15 ml)
6	large medjool dates, chopped
	or
1/2 cup	carob chips (125ml)
	or
1/2 cup	raisins (125 ml)

These muffins are so simple to make and very tasty, especially if you use big, juicy dates.

- Oil muffin tins.

- In a large bowl, mash bananas and add water. Add oil and syrup. Add all dry ingredients and mix well. If using carob chips, stir in; if not, add in dates.

- Spoon into prepared muffin tins and bake at 375F for 15-18 minutes. Cool for 5 minutes and remove from muffin tins.

If you use brown rice flour and spelt, you may need to add a bit more water, as the muffin mix may be too dry. You want the mixture to be sticky and clumpy.

If you use raisins or dates instead of carob chips, you can omit the sweetener, as the dates will sweeten the muffins naturally.

Yields 12 muffins. These muffins freeze well.

NOTE
You can purchase vitamin C crystals and guar gum at your local health food store. Try spelt, kamut, barley, brown rice, or quinoa flour in this recipe.

Blueberry Banana Muffins

Free of dairy products, wheat, yeast, corn, sugar, eggs, soy, nuts, nightshades, and gluten.

Ingredients

3/4 cup	chickpea flour (175 ml)
1/4 cup	arrowroot flour (50 ml)
1/4 cup	tapioca flour (50 ml)
1/4 cup	potato starch (50 ml)
1/2 cup	brown rice flour (125 ml)
2 tsp	baking soda (10 ml)
1 tsp	xanthan gum or guar gum (5 ml)
2 tsp	cinnamon (10 ml)
1 tsp	vanilla (5 ml)
1/4 cup	maple syrup (50 ml)
1/2 cup	safflower oil (125 ml)
1/4 cup	water (50 ml)
4	bananas, mashed
1 cup	blueberries (250 ml)

- Mash bananas in a bowl with water.
- Add oil, maple syrup, and vanilla and mix well.
- Add in remaining ingredients and mix.
- Spoon into muffin tins and bake at 350F for approximately 30 minutes.

Yields 12 muffins.

NOTE

If you want these muffins to be corn-free, use guar gum instead of xanthan gum.

Apple Walnut Muffins

Free of dairy products, wheat, yeast, sugar, eggs, soy, nuts, nightshades, and gluten.

- In your food processor mix banana, apple, apple juice, and walnuts.

- Pour mixture into a mixing bowl and add remaining ingredients.

- Mix well and spoon into muffin tins and bake at 350 F for 30 minutes or until done.

Yields 12 muffins.

Ingredients

3/4 cup	chickpea flour (175 ml)
1/4 cup	arrowroot flour (50 ml)
1/4 cup	tapioca flour (50 ml)
1/4 cup	potato starch (50 ml)
1/2 cup	brown rice flour (125 ml)
2 tsp	baking soda (10 ml)
1 tsp	xanthan gum or guar gum (5 ml)
2 tsp	cinnamon (10 ml)
1 tsp	nutmeg (5 ml)
1 1/2 cups	apple juice (375 ml)
2	apples, diced
1	banana, mashed
1 cup	walnuts (250 ml)

NOTE

If you want these muffins to be corn-free, use guar gum instead of xanthan gum.

Peanut Butter Banana Muffins

Free of dairy products, wheat, yeast, sugar, eggs, soy, nightshades, and gluten.

Ingredients

3	bananas, mashed
1/4 cup	water (50 ml)
1/2 cup	safflower oil (125 ml)
1 cup	crunchy peanut butter (250 ml)
1/4 cup	maple syrup (50 ml)
3/4 cup	chickpea flour (175 ml)
1/4 cup	arrowroot flour (50 ml)
1/4 cup	tapioca flour (50 ml)
1/4 cup	potato starch (50 ml)
1/2 cup	brown rice flour (125 ml)
2 tsp	baking soda (10 ml)
1 tsp	xanthan gum (5 ml)

- Mash bananas in a bowl with water and oil. Mix in peanut butter and maple syrup. Add in flours and mix well.

- Spoon into muffin tins and bake at 350F for 30 minutes.

Yields 12 muffins.

Sweet Potato Dessert

Free of wheat, yeast, corn, sugar, eggs, soy, nightshades, and gluten. If you want this to be dairy-free, use oil instead of butter.

Ingredients

2	cups sweet potatoes, diced (2 small sweet potatoes or 1 large one) (500 ml)
1/3 cup	coconut oil or butter (75 ml)
1 cup	rice or nut milk (250 ml)
3/4 cup	raisins (175 ml)
1 tsp	cardamom (5 ml)
1 tsp	cinnamon (5 ml)
1/2 cup	ground almonds (125 ml)

- In a pan, cook sweet potato in oil for a few minutes to soften the potato; stir frequently.

- In a large casserole dish, mix sweet potato-oil mixture, rice milk, raisins, cardamom, cinnamon, and almonds.

- Bake in 400F oven for approximately 30-40 minutes.

  You can modify this recipe by leaving out the nuts and adding unsweetened coconut, if you prefer.

Yields 3 cups (750 ml).

DID YOU KNOW?

This large edible root is from the morning glory family.

There are many varieties of sweet potato but the two that are popular are the pale sweet potato and the darker-skinned variety, which is often called the "yam." The true yam is not related to the sweet potato.

Lemon Almond Biscotti

Free of dairy products, wheat, yeast, corn, sugar, soy, and nightshades.

Ingredients

1 3/4 cups	spelt flour (425 ml)
1/4 cup	maple syrup, honey, rice malt, or barley malt (50 ml)
1 cup	whole raw almonds, coarsely ground in food processor (250 ml)
	Zest of 1 organic lemon, grated
1 Tbsp	baking powder (15 ml)
1/3 cup	safflower oil (75 ml)
2	organic eggs
1 tsp	pure vanilla extract (5 ml)
1 tsp	pure almond extract (5 ml)
	Juice of 1 lemon

- Grind nuts in your food processor until fine. Place nuts in a large mixing bowl. Stir in flour, lemon zest, and baking powder.

- If you have a food processor, throw all wet ingredients into it and mix well. If not, mix all wet ingredients in a separate bowl: oil, egg or flax mixture, vanilla, almond extract, sweetener, and lemon juice. Mix your dry ingredients and wet ingredients.

- Preheat oven to 325F.

- Line baking dish or cookie sheet with parchment paper (wet one side of parchment paper, that side down); this helps maintain moisture without its being soggy. If you do not have parchment paper, oil and flour your pan.

- With greased hands or an oiled spatula, flatten out mixture. You want it quite thin for biscotti.

- Drop pan on counter twice, this helps to settle it.

Lemon Almond Biscotti

- Bake 30 minutes on top oven rack, but check at 20 minutes if cooking with spelt flour, as it cooks faster than wheat flour.

- When golden, take out of the oven. Let it cool for 20 minutes and then cut into squares with sharp spatula.

  If you use a knife, you will cut your parchment paper and will not be able to reuse it.

Yields 1 small-size cookie sheet.

NOTE

I have made this recipe using flaxseed mixture or tofu as substitutes for eggs. Both work, but biscotti will not be as light and fluffy if you substitute out the eggs.

Banana Date Cookies

Free of dairy products, wheat, yeast, corn, sugar, eggs, soy, and nightshades. This can be made nut free if you omit the walnuts.

Ingredients

3	ripe bananas
1 cup	dates, chopped, or carob chips (250 ml)
1/2 cup	walnuts (optional) (125 ml)
1/3 cup	olive oil (75 ml)
1 tsp	pure vanilla (5 ml)
2 cups	rolled oats (500 ml)
1 Tbsp	honey (optional) (15 ml)

- In a bowl, mash bananas and add everything else. Let mixture stand for 20 minutes to let oats absorb moisture. Shape into rounds on cookie sheet.

- Bake at 400F for 20 minutes.

Yields 20 cookies.

NOTE

You can also use carob chips instead of dates and you can omit the nuts if you like.

Try barley flakes or kamut flakes instead of oat flakes if you have a problem with oats.

DID YOU KNOW?

Dates go back over years with the name coming from the Greek word Daktulos, meaning "finger" after the shape of the fruit. They are a good source of protein and iron, so enjoy these cookies, they are good for you!

Fruit and Nut Bars

Free of dairy products, wheat, yeast, corn, sugar, eggs, soy, nightshades, and gluten.

These are great! Fast and easy, and a real treat.

- Place almonds, raisins, dates and lemon peel in food processor. Using the blender blade, process mixture, grinding it finely.

- Sprinkle the bottom of an 8X8-inch cake pan with half the coconut.

- Using your hands, evenly press fruit nut mixture over the coconut to cover the bottom of the pan.

- Sprinkle the remainder of the coconut on top.

- Chill the mixture for 2 hours, then cut into bars and enjoy.

Ingredients

1 cup	whole raw almonds (250 ml)
1 cup	raisins (250 ml)
1 cup	pitted dates (250 ml)
	Rind of 1 lemon, grated
1/3 cup	shredded, unsweetened coconut (75 ml)

Gingerbread Cookies

Free of dairy products, wheat, yeast, corn, sugar, eggs, soy, and nightshades.

Ingredients

1/2 cup	barley flour (125 ml)
1/2 cup	brown rice flour (125 ml)
1/2 tsp	cream of tartar (2 ml)
1/2 tsp	baking soda (2 ml)
1 Tbsp	freshly grated ginger, or more if you really want them to be gingery (15 ml)
1/2 cup	ground pecans (125 ml)
1-2 Tbsp	honey or maple syrup (15-30 ml)
4 Tbsp	orange juice (60 ml)
	Zest of 1 orange, grated

- Grind the pecans to a fine dust, using your food processor. The mixture should be oily.

- Add the dry ingredients, then add wet ingredients; mix well in food processor.

- Roll cookies into small balls and flatten out into cookies with a fork (like peanut butter cookies) or roll out dough thinly on a floured board and cut into cookie shapes or into cute little men, or whatever shape the kids like.

- Cook on a lightly greased tray and bake 15-20 minutes at 350F.

Yields 16 small cookies.

Birthday Cake

Free of dairy products, wheat, yeast, corn, sugar, eggs, soy, nuts, nightshades, and gluten. If you use spelt or kamut then it will have gluten.

- Mix dry ingredients in a bowl.

- Mix wet ingredients in a bowl.

- Add wet to dry and stir. Your mixture will bubble, due to the vinegar and soda reacting together.

- Stir well and spoon into an oiled 8x8-inch cake pan immediately or mixture will go stiff.

- Bake at 375F for 18-20 minutes.

  Top with any of the icings offered in this cookbook.

Yields 1 cake.

Ingredients

3 cups	brown rice flour, spelt flour, or kamut flour (750 ml)
1/2 cup	unsweetened carob or cocoa powder (125ml)
2 tsp	baking soda (10 ml)
2 tsp	baking powder (10 ml)
1 tsp	vitamin C crystals (5 ml)
1/2 tsp	guar gum (2 ml)
1-1 1/2 cups	warm water* (250-375 ml)
1/4-1/2 cup	maple syrup (50-125 ml)
2 Tbsp	apple cider vinegar (30 ml)
2 tsp	pure vanilla (10 ml)
4 Tbsp	safflower or coconut oil (60 ml)
1/2 cup	apple butter (125ml)

* Amount of water will depend on which flour you are using.

NOTE

This is a great recipe for your child if he or she has allergies to wheat, Dairy, eggs, or gluten. It is also low in sugar; most birthday cakes are full of refined sugar.

You can also make this recipe into cupcakes and ice them individually.

For a nice gluten free cake try using Bob's Red Mill gluten-free flour mix.

Pseudo-Brownies

Free of dairy products, wheat, yeast, corn, sugar, eggs, soy, nightshades, and gluten.

Ingredients

1 cup	brown rice flour (250 ml)
1/4 cup	carob or cocoa powder (50 ml)
1	heaping tsp baking soda
2 tsp	cream of tartar (10 ml)
1	large organic apple, peeled and chopped
1/2 cup	raisins (125 ml)
1/2 cup	chopped walnuts or pecans (125 ml)
2 Tbsp	honey (optional) (30 ml)
2	eggs or substitute (2 heaping Tbsp [30 ml] flaxseed with 3/4 cup [175 ml] water. Bring to a boil and let cool.)
2 Tbsp	apple butter (30 ml)

This is a very easy recipe and I feel everyone needs a brownie in his/her life now and then. I refused to believe that since I had allergies, I would never eat a brownie again; hence this recipe.

- All I do is grab my food processor and throw in raisins, nuts, a cut-up, peeled apple, and mix.

- Then I add in honey if I am using any, eggs or flaxseed mixture, and mix again.

- Then I add carob powder, rice flour, baking soda, and cream of tartar and mix until all is combined. If it seems dry, I add a drop or two of water.

- Finally, I place mix in an 8-inch square brownie pan and bake at 350F for 20-25 minutes.

  Eat as is, or top with brownie icing.

NOTE

I have also made these brownies with spelt and quinoa flour and cocoa instead of carob. Both work well.

Pseudo-Brownie Icing

Free of dairy products, wheat, yeast, corn, sugar, eggs, soy, nightshades, and gluten.

Ingredients

1/2 cup	cashew butter (125 ml)
4 Tbsp	maple syrup (60 ml)
1/2 tsp	vanilla (2 ml)
2 Tbsp	carob or cocoa powder (30 ml)
2 Tbsp	orange juice (30 ml)
	or
1-2 Tbsp	hot water (optional) (15-30 ml)

- Place all ingredients in a bowl and stir until smooth.
- Add liquids slowly, as you do not want to make this icing too liquidy.

Good for cake or brownie icing.

Yields 1/2 cup (125 ml).

NOTE

If your cashew butter is runny, you may not need any liquid. Also try macadamia nut butter instead of cashew butter. You can also substitute cocoa for carob if you prefer.

Date and Carob Icing

Free of dairy products, wheat, yeast, corn, sugar, eggs, soy, nuts, nightshades, and gluten.

Ingredients

1/2 cup	chopped dates (125 ml)
2 Tbsp	carob powder (30 ml)
2-3 Tbsp	boiling water (30-45 ml)
3 Tbsp	maple syrup (45 ml)
1 tsp	orange rind (5 ml)
1 Tbsp	orange juice (15 ml)
	Shredded unsweetened coconut or chopped nuts for decoration (optional)

- Mash dates and pour boiling water over them. Mix in remaining ingredients except for coconut or nuts.

- Blend until smooth.

Yields 1/2 cup (125 ml).

Carob Tahini Icing

Free of dairy products, wheat, yeast, corn, sugar, eggs, soy, nuts, nightshades, and gluten. This recipe can be nut free if you use soy milk or rice milk.

- Blend all ingredients in a bowl and chill in refrigerator for at least 2 hours. Use as a cream over fruit or on pies.

  I love to drizzle this over my strawberry fruit mousse; it is to die for and a real treat.

  You can use water instead of the milk, but expect it to be a different consistency.

Yields 3/4 cup (175 ml).

NOTE

If your tahini is soft, you may not need to add any liquid.

Ingredients

1/4 cup	tahini (50 ml)
1/8 cup	nut, soy, or rice milk (25 ml)
1 tsp	vanilla (5 ml)
1/4 cup	honey or maple syrup (50 ml)
1 Tbsp	carob powder (15 ml)

Carrot Date Muffins

Free of dairy products, wheat, yeast, corn, sugar, eggs, soy, nuts, and nightshades.

Ingredients

2/3 cup	safflower or coconut oil (150 ml)
1/4 cup	honey (optional) (50 ml)
2 cups	unsweetened applesauce (500 ml)
1/2 cup	flaxseed mixture (125 ml) (6 Tbsp [90 ml] water with 2 Tbsp [30 ml] ground flaxseed. Blend in blender until frothy or with a whisk.)
2/3 cup	chopped dates (150 ml)
2 cups	carrots, grated (500 ml)
1 tsp	nutmeg (5 ml)
2 tsp	cinnamon (10 ml)
2 tsp	baking soda (10 ml)
4 tsp	baking powder (20 ml)
3-4 cups	spelt flour, or oat, barley or kamut flour (750 ml-1 L)

- Grate carrots in your food processor.

- Mix grated carrots, applesauce, and oil together in a bowl. Add in flaxseed mixture, which replaces an egg. Add nutmeg, cinnamon, baking soda, and baking powder, and then add your flour slowly. You may need all 4 cups, depending on the type of flour you are using.

- Mix in cut-up dates and mix well.

- Spoon into muffin tins and bake at 350F for 30 minutes or until golden brown.

You can add more dates and leave out the honey if you want to cut down on sugar content. Or you can use Stevia to sweeten, as it has no calories, does not affect your blood sugar, and is natural. See note on sugar substitutes at front of book for more info.

Yields 16 muffins.

NOTE

These muffins are great but a little more time-consuming to make than the banana Date muffins. I usually use oat or spelt flour in this recipe, but you can also use brown rice flour.

Cranberry Loaf

Free of dairy products, wheat, yeast, corn, sugar, eggs, soy, nuts, and nightshades.

- Mix dry ingredients together in a bowl, then cut in oil until mixture is crumbly. Add in egg or flaxseed mixture, orange peel, and juice all at once. Stir until mixture is moist. Fold in cranberries and raisins.

- Spoon into greased 8 1/2-inch (1.5 L) loaf pan and bake at 350F for 1 hour.

Yields 1 loaf.

Delicious at Christmastime or in the Autumn when there is a nip in the air. Lovely to have a slice of this with a nice cup of herbal tea.

NOTE
I also make this recipe using oat or kamut flour. For a gluten-free loaf try using Bob's Red Mill gluten-free flour mix.

Ingredients

2 cups	spelt flour (500 ml)
1/4 cup	maple syrup (50 ml)
1 1/2 tsp	baking powder (7 ml)
1/2 tsp	baking soda (2 ml)
1 tsp	sea salt (5 ml)
1/2 cup	oil (125 ml)
1	egg, beaten, or use flaxseed mixture (2 Tbsp [30 ml] ground flaxseed and 6 Tbsp [90 ml] water, mix in blender and use instead of egg)
1-2 tsp	grated orange rind (5-10 ml)
1/2 tsp	grated lemon zest (2 ml)
3/4 cup	orange juice (175 ml)
1 cup	raisins (250 ml)
1 cup	fresh cranberries (250 ml)

Sweet Potato Muffins

Free of dairy products, wheat, yeast, corn, sugar, eggs, soy, nightshades, and gluten.

Ingredients

3⁄4 cup	chickpea flour (175 ml)
3⁄4 cup	brown rice flour (175 ml)
1⁄4 cup	tapioca flour (50 ml)
1⁄4 cup	potato starch (50 ml)
2 tbsp	hemp seed (30 ml)
1 tsp	baking powder (5 ml)
1 tsp	baking soda (5 ml)
1 tsp	cinnamon (5 ml)
1⁄2 tsp	nutmeg (2 ml)
1⁄2 tsp	sea salt (2 ml)
1 1⁄2 cup	mashed cooked sweet potato (375 ml)
1 tsp	pure vanilla extract (5 ml)
1/3 cup	canola, safflower, or coconut oil (75 ml)
1/3 cup	organic coconut milk (75 ml)
1/4 cup	maple syrup (50 ml)
1/2 cup	pecans (125 ml)

- Mix all dry ingredients together.
- Add in wet ingredient and mix well. Stir in nuts.
- Fill muffin tins and bake 350F for 25 mins or until done.

Yields 12 muffins.

Fruit Mousse

Free of dairy products, wheat, yeast, corn, sugar, eggs, nuts, nightshades, and gluten.

Ingredients

3 cups	fresh strawberry pulp or any other fruit of your choice (750 ml)
1 cup	almond milk or soy milk (250 ml)
2-3 Tbsp	agar flakes (30-45 ml)
1/2 cup	water (125 ml)
	Juice of 2 lemons
2 Tbsp	honey (30 ml)

- Blend strawberries or fruit of your choice with milk in a blender or food processor to make pulp.

- In a saucepan, place water, agar flakes, lemon juice, and honey. Bring to a boil and then reduce to simmer for a few minutes until agar has dissolved.

- Remove from heat and let stand for a few minutes to cool down a bit and then add to fruit pulp and mix.

- Pour into glass dessert bowls and refrigerate.

  Serve chilled with a strawberry on top or drizzle carob tahini icing on top. See page 183.

  If your fruit is not in season and not that sweet, you may have to add a bit more honey.

Yields 4 cups (1 L).

NOTE

Agar is sometimes difficult to work with. It makes things jell, so you would use it instead of gelatin. Sometimes when I make this recipe I add 2 Tbsp (30 mL) of agar and put it in the fridge only to see it set right away. Other times I will look in the fridge 2 hours later and it is still a bit on the runny side. If you are new at using agar, you will have to experiment with it a bit. Even if your mousse is a bit runny, call it pudding instead; it still will be delicious!

Carob Banana Pie

Free of dairy products, wheat, yeast, corn, sugar, eggs, soy, nightshades, and gluten.

Ingredients

Crust:

3/4 cup	almonds (175 ml)
3/4 cup	brown rice flour (175 ml)
1/3 cup	safflower or coconut oil (75 ml)
1/8 cup	maple syrup (25 ml)
	Pinch sea salt
1/4 tsp	cinnamon (1 ml)

Filling:

4 cups	carob rice milk (1 L)
1/4 cup	agar flakes (50 ml)
1/4 cup	maple syrup (50 ml)
1/3-1/2 cup	arrowroot flour (75-125 ml)
1 tsp	pure vanilla extract (5 ml)
2-3	bananas, sliced

Crust:

- Soak almonds for 2 hours in a bowl full of water. Rinse and dry almonds before grinding them.

- In a food processor, grind almonds until they are relatively fine. Add rice flour, salt, and cinnamon, and mix until combined. Then add in oil and maple syrup and mix well.

- Press mixture into a 10-inch pie plate and bake at 350F for 25 minutes or until brown. Let pie crust cool.

Filling:

- Bring rice milk and agar to a boil and then simmer until agar has dissolved.

- In a separate bowl or measuring cup, mix arrowroot and maple syrup and then whisk it into the rice milk. The mixture should thicken right away. Remove from stove, and allow it to cool for 20 minutes. When ready, slice bananas into the cooled pie shell and then pour the rice milk mixture over the bananas and place in fridge to cool.

  It will congeal in the fridge and is a lovely, light dessert. You can substitute cocoa for carob.

Yields 1 pie.

NOTE
Sometimes carob rice milk is hard to find. You can make your own by using plain rice milk and adding in carob powder or cocoa powder (1/4 cup or 50 mL).

Sunflower Oat Bars

Free of dairy products, wheat, yeast, corn, sugar, eggs, soy, nuts, nightshades and gluten.

- In a food processor, grind oats, apple, and dates. Add a little hot water to help combine the ingredients. Then add the remaining ingredients and combine well. If it is to dry, add a little more water so it is pasty.

- Let mixture sit for 10 minutes.

- Spread mixture into a lightly greased 8-inch square dish and bake at 350F for 25 minutes or until done.

- Cut into squares when cool.

Yields 1 pan.

Ingredients

2 cups	gluten-free rolled oats (1 cup to be blended finely) (500ml)
4-5 Tbsp	sunflower seeds (60-75 ml)
2 Tbsp	pepitas (pumpkin seeds) (30 ml)
1/4 tsp	sea salt (1 ml)
1	apple, grated
	Zest of 1 lemon, grated
6	large dates, chopped finely
2 Tbsp	coconut oil (30 ml)
	Boiling water

Apple Crisp

Free of dairy products, wheat, yeast, corn, sugar, eggs, soy, nuts, nightshades and gluten.

Ingredients

6-8	organic apples, sliced
2 tsp	cinnamon (10 ml)

Topping:

2/3 cup	flour (oat, spelt, barley, or kamut flour) (150 ml)
2 cups	flakes (oat, barley, kamut, or spelt) (500 ml)
2/3 cup	coconut oil, butter or margarine (150ml)
1/4-1/2 cup	maple syrup, honey, or rice syrup (50-125 ml)

- Put apples in a lightly greased 8-inch square baking dish, sprinkle with cinnamon, and mix.

- In a bowl, mix flour, oats, coconut oil, and sweetener. Knead with hands to make topping crumbly.

- Spread this mixture over the apples and bake at 375F until golden for 30-40 minutes.

  This can be gluten-free if you used gluten free oats and gluten free oat flour

Yields 1 pan.

Strawberry Hemp Ice

Free of dairy products, wheat, yeast, corn, sugar, eggs, soy, nuts, nightshades, and gluten.

Ingredients

1 cup	hulled hemp seed (washed) (250 ml)
1 cup	frozen or fresh strawberries (250 ml)
1 Tbsp	maple syrup or honey (15 ml)
1/4 tsp	guar gum (1 ml)
1/2	banana

- In food processor, mix strawberries and maple syrup, then add hemp, guar gum, and banana and mix well until hemp seeds are processed. If you like a crunchy taste, do not mix as long.

- Put in small containers and put in freezer.

  For a smoother texture, add a bit of coconut milk.

  Enjoy, and no, this ice cream will not make you high!

Yields 2 cups (500 ml).

Carob Banana Hemp Ice

Free of dairy products, wheat, yeast, corn, sugar, eggs, soy, nuts, nightshades, and gluten.

Ingredients

3/4 cup	shelled hemp seeds (washed) (175 ml)
3	bananas, mashed
1-2 Tbsp	maple syrup (15-30 ml)
1-2 Tbsp	unsweetened carob powder (15-30 ml)
1/4 tsp	guar gum (1 ml)
3/4 cup	coconut milk (175 ml)

- Mix all ingredients together in food processor for at least 10 minutes to break up the hemp.

- Dish small amounts into containers and place in the freezer.

  Take out of freezer 5 minutes before you wish to eat it, so that it softens a bit.

Yields 3 cups (750 ml).

NOTE

You can use unsweetened organic cocoa instead of carob for a yummy, healthy chocolate dessert.

Oatmeal Cookies

Free of wheat, yeast, corn, sugar, eggs, soy, nuts, nightshades and gluten.

- Mix butter and honey together. Add egg, vanilla, and water and mix well. Then add remaining ingredients and mix.

  For a change, you can also add a sprinkling of cinnamon and nutmeg to this recipe.

- Spoon drops onto cookie sheet and bake at 375F for 10-12 minutes, and voilà, oatmeal cookies!

Yields 18 small cookies.

Ingredients

3 Tbsp	butter (45 ml)
3 Tbsp	honey (45 ml)
1	egg or egg replacer
1/3 cup	water (75 ml)
1 tsp	vanilla (5 ml)
1 tsp	almond extract (optional) (5 ml)
1/4 cup	gluten-free oat flour (50ml)
1/2 tsp	baking powder (2 ml)
1/2 cup	ground sunflower seeds (125 ml)
3/4 cup	gluten-free rolled oats (175ml)
1/2 cup	raisins or (125 ml)
1/2 cup	carob chips (125 ml)

If you can't use butter, try using margarine or coconut oil in this recipe

Lime Coconut Cookies

Free of dairy products, wheat, yeast, corn, sugar, eggs, soy, nuts, nightshades, and gluten.

Ingredients

1 cup	brown rice flour (250 ml)
1/4 cup	tapioca flour (50 ml)
1/4 cup	potato flour (50 ml)
1 Tbsp	ground flaxseed (15 ml) mixed with 3 Tbsp (45 ml) water in blender (egg replacer)
1 cup	shredded unsweetened coconut (250 ml)
1/3 cup	rice syrup (75 ml)
	Zest of 1 lime
	Juice of 2 limes
1/3 cup	safflower oil or macadamia nut oil (75 ml)
1/4 tsp	almond oil (1 ml) or 1/2 tsp (2 ml) vanilla

- Mix brown rice flour, tapioca, and potato flour together in a bowl with a whisk.

- In a separate bowl, mix oil, rice syrup, flaxseed mixture, zest and juice of limes, and almond oil.

- Now mix wet ingredients in with dry. Add in shredded coconut and mix with your hands. Shape into rounds and place on a greased cookie sheet and bake at 350F for 10-15 minutes or until done.

  This is a gluten-free cookie, so it will be a bit crumbly due to the flours used.

Yields 16 cookies.

NOTE

A hint when using rice syrup: Measure out your oil first, then your syrup, as it will pour out of your measuring cup much easier if your cup is still coated with a bit of oil.

Christmas Treats

Free of dairy products, wheat, yeast, corn, sugar, eggs, soy, nightshades, and gluten.

- Chop apricots and dates into pieces and place in a saucepan with orange juice, water, and honey. Cover and simmer over low to medium heat until fruit is tender and liquid has evaporated. This should take about 5-10 minutes.

- Remove from heat and let fruit cool.

- Purée fruit in a food processor until it is pasty. Add zest and nuts and mix in a bowl.

- With slightly oiled fingers, pinch off a small amount and roll into balls and coat with coconut.

- Place on a tray and let sit in a cool place for a day, and then enjoy.

  If you are watching your sugar intake, you do not have to add honey to this recipe, as the apricots and dates will make it quite sweet.

Yields 18 small balls.

Ingredients

1/2 cup	dried apricots (125 ml)
1/2 cup	dates (125 ml)
2 Tbsp	orange juice (30 ml)
2 Tbsp	honey (30 ml)
3 Tbsp	water (45 ml)
1 tsp	orange rind or lemon zest (5 ml)
1/4 cup	pecans, chopped finely (50 ml)
3/4 cup	shredded unsweetened coconut (175 ml)

Christmas Cashew Balls

Free of dairy products, wheat, yeast, corn, sugar, eggs, soy, nightshades, and gluten.

Ingredients

1 cup	unsalted cashew pieces (250 ml)
1/8 tsp	ground cardamom (.5 ml)
1 cup	dates, finely chopped (250 ml)
	Zest of 1 orange
1 Tbsp	orange juice (15 ml)
1/2 cup	shredded unsweetened coconut (125 ml)

- Roast your cashew pieces in a cast-iron pan, but stir often so they do not burn. It will take only a few minutes to get a nice roasted flavour, or you can cheat and buy roasted cashews.

- Grind cashews in a food processor but not too finely. Add in cardamom, dates, orange peel, and orange juice and mix.

- Roll into small balls, then roll in coconut. Eat and enjoy! No baking needed.

Yields 18 balls.

Orange Teff Cookies

Free of dairy products, wheat, yeast, corn, sugar, eggs, soy, nightshades and gluten.

Ingredients

1 1/3 cups	teff flour (325 ml)
2 cups	almonds (500 ml)
2 cups	gluten-free rolled oats (500ml)
1 tsp	ground nutmeg (5 ml)
1/4 tsp	sea salt (1 ml)
2/3 cup	safflower oil (150 ml)
1/4 cup	maple syrup (50 ml)
1 tsp	vanilla (5 ml)
1/2 cup	orange juice (125 ml)
	Rind of 1 orange
2/3 cup	unsweetened applesauce (150 ml)

- In a food processor, grind the almonds and the oats until relatively fine.

- Place in a bowl. Add flour, nutmeg, and salt and mix well.

- In another bowl, mix oil, maple syrup, orange juice, rind, and vanilla. Mix dry ingredients into wet, and mix well. If the mixture is too dry, add a bit more orange juice or some water.

  This mixture can be very dry with the teff and the almonds. You want to be able to roll balls of dough in your hands without it crumbling.

- Roll into balls and flatten onto cookie sheet with a fork to make cookies.

- Bake at 325F for approximately 20-25 minutes, depending on your oven.

Yields 30 small cookies.

DID YOU KNOW?

Teff is an ancient grain grown in Africa. It has been grown in Ethiopia for eons and is high in protein and carbohydrates and a good source of calcium and iron.

Teff Peanut Butter Cookies

Free of dairy products, wheat, yeast, corn, sugar, eggs, soy, nightshades, and gluten.

Ingredients

1 1/2 cups	teff flour (375 ml)
1/4 cup	maple syrup (50 ml)
1/2 cup	safflower or coconut oil (125 ml)
1 tsp	pure vanilla extract (5 ml)
1 cup	crunchy peanut butter, cashew butter, or almond butter (250 ml)
1/4 tsp	sea salt (1 ml)

- In a food processor, mix peanut butter, oil, maple syrup, and vanilla but do not overmix. Then add in teff flour and salt and mix together. The mixture should just stick together and roll into balls nicely.

- Shape into balls and place on cookie sheet and flatten gently with wet fork.

- Bake at 350F for 10-15 minutes.

  These cookies are very yummy but a bit crumbly.

Yields 24 cookies.

NOTE

Try adding in 3/4 cup (175 mL) of gluten-free cereal for a crunchier cookie. I buy a buckwheat flake cereal by Arrowhead Mills and add it in. Or try amaranth flakes.

Rice Pudding with Lemon

Free of dairy products, wheat, yeast, corn, sugar, eggs, soy, nuts, nightshades, and gluten.

Ingredients

1 cup	coconut milk (250 ml)
1 cup	water (250 ml)
1/2 cup	organic long grain white rice (125 ml)
1 Tbsp	honey (15 ml)
1/4 tsp	sea salt (1 ml)
1 tsp	pure vanilla extract (5 ml)
	Juice and zest of half a lemon

- In a pot, combine coconut milk, water, salt, vanilla, and rice. Bring to a boil and then reduce to low, cover, and cook for 30 minutes. Stir occasionally. Add honey at the end of cooking.

- Remove from heat and stir in lemon juice and zest and place in a bowl in the fridge for 1 hour before serving.

You can top this with fresh fruit or toasted coconut.

Yields 2 cups (500 ml).

Barley Pudding

Free of dairy products, wheat, yeast, corn, sugar, eggs, soy, nuts, and nightshades.

Ingredients

1 1/2 cups	cooked pearl barley (375 ml)
1/4 cup	Thompson raisins (50 ml)
2 cups	coconut milk (500 ml)
1/8 tsp	cinnamon (.5 ml)
	Sprinkle of nutmeg, cinnamon, and cardamom
1 tsp	maple syrup (5 ml)

- Place cooked barley, raisins, milk, cinnamon, and maple syrup in a clay pot or casserole dish with a lid. Sprinkle mixture of nutmeg, cinnamon, and cardamom on top and bake at 350F for 1 hour.

If too dry, add more milk and return to oven.

Yields 2 servings.

Carrot Haystacks

Free of dairy products, wheat, yeast, corn, sugar, eggs, soy, nuts, nightshades, and gluten.

- In a bowl, mix shredded carrots, sea salt, safflower oil, flour, coconut, and honey. Mix ground flaxseed in 6 tablespoons of water and whisk to make an egg-like consistency; mix in with carrot mixture.

- Mix water and arrowroot together and mix with other ingredients.

- Mix all together, mould into small shapes onto baking sheet and bake at 325F for 10-15 minutes or until done.

Yields 16 cookies.

Ingredients

1 cup	carrots, shredded (250 ml)
2 1/2 cups	shredded unsweetened coconut (625 ml)
2 Tbsp	cold water (30 ml)
2 Tbsp	arrowroot powder (30 ml)
2 Tbsp	coconut oil (30 ml)
3 Tbsp	honey (45 ml)
2 Tbsp	ground flaxseed (30 ml) and 6 Tbsp (90 ml) water (whisked)
2 Tbsp	brown rice flour (30 ml)
	Pinch sea salt

Carob Haystacks

Free of dairy products, wheat, yeast, corn, sugar, eggs, soy, nuts, nightshades, and gluten.

Ingredients

1/4 cup	carob powder* (50 ml)
2 cups	shredded unsweetened coconut (500 ml)
2 Tbsp	cold water (30 ml)
2 Tbsp	arrowroot (30 ml)
2 Tbsp	coconut oil (30 ml)
4 Tbsp	honey (60 ml)
2 Tbsp	ground flaxseed (30 ml) and 6 Tbsp (90 ml) water (whisked)
	Pinch salt

* You can use organic unsweetened cocoa instead of carob powder.

- In a bowl or food processor, mix water, arrowroot, and carob powder. Mix well so ingredients dissolve and mixture is smooth.

- Add in remaining ingredients.

- Mould into round shapes onto cookie sheet and bake at 325F for 10-15 minutes or until done.

  I like this recipe, as you can make these haystacks as sweet as you like. If you like them sweet, add in more honey or use sweetened coconut. If you are like me and don't like things sweet, leave as is.

Yields 12 cookies.

Cashew Muffins

Free of dairy products, wheat, yeast, corn, sugar, eggs, soy, and nightshades.

- Mix dry ingredients in a bowl.

- In a food processor, blend banana, apple juice, apple, and cashews. It is nice to leave a few small chunks of apple, so do not blend too well.

- Mix wet with dry and pour into lightly oiled muffin tins two-thirds full.

- Bake 35-45 minutes at 325F.

Yields 12 muffins.

NOTE
TRY using 1 cup brown rice and 1 cup quinoa flour for a nice gluten-free muffin.

Ingredients

1 cup	spelt flour (250 ml)
1 cup	brown rice flour (250 ml)
1 1/2 cups	unsweetened apple juice (375 ml)
1	organic apple, peeled and chopped
2	ripe bananas
1/2 cup	chopped cashews (125 ml)
4 tsp	baking powder (20 ml)
1 1/2 tsp	cinnamon (7 ml)
1/2 tsp	nutmeg (2 ml)

Food Families

Alphabetical

Introduction

Deprived of things to eat? Here is a comprehensive list of foods from A to Z and the number of the family to which each belongs so it will be easier for you to plan your rotation diet.

We tend to restrict our diets to a small percentage of foods. Treat your allergy as a challenge. Use the lists that follow to try new possibilities.

How to use these charts:

List 1 is an alphabetical list of foods. The number preceding each item indicates the food family to which it belongs. List 2 is food families in numerical order.

For example, let's say you are allergic to cucumbers. You need to know whether or not there are other members of the same family that may cause you reactions. In front of "cucumber" in List 1 is the number 29. If you turn to number 29 on List 2 you will see a list of foods that is part of the whole food family, the Gourd family. Pumpkins, squash, and cantaloupe are members of this family, so you may need to avoid these as well.

When you are planning your rotation diet you must pay attention to food families until you know what foods you are reacting to. Some people are so allergic that they may do well to avoid all foods pertaining to the food family that they are reacting to. Others will be fine avoiding only the foods that present them with problems.

A

107	abalone	42	althea root	66b	apricot	5	arrowroot (Musa)
38	acacia (gum)	2	amaranth	73	arrowroot (Brazilian, tapioca)	13	arrowroot, Queensland
43	acerola	3	amaryllis	4	arrowroot (Colocasia)	18	artichoke flour
29	acorn squash	103	amberjack	26	arrowroot, East Indian (Curcuma)	4	Arum Family
1	agar agar	94	american eel			39	asparagus
3	agave	81	anchovy	75	arrowroot, Fiji (tacca)	37	avocado
104	albacore	16	angelica	21	arrowroot, Florida (Zamia)		
38	alfalfa	16	anise				
1	algae	8	annatto				
49	allspice	113	antelope				
66b	almond	66a	apple				
39	aloe vera	45	apple mint				

25	baker's yeast	85	beef	18	boneset	48	Brussel sprout
31	bamboo shoots	28	beet	104	bonito	10	buckwheat
5	banana	63	bell pepper	9	borage	85	buffalo
43	Barbados cherry	45	bergamot	29	Boston marrow	31	bulgur
31	barley	7	Birch Family	85	Bovine Family	18	burdock root
45	basil	8	Bixa Family	66c	boysenberry	66b	burnet
127	bass (black)	66c	blackberry	31	bran	11	Buttercup Family
82	bass (yellow)	38	black-eyed peas	30	brandy	29	buttercup squash
40	basswood	59	black pepper	73	Brazilian	100	butterfish
37	bay leaf	18	black salsify		arrowroot	79	butternut
38	bean	79	black walnut	69	Brazil nut	29	butternut squash
83	bear	32	blueberry	47	breadfruit		
32	bearberry	84	bluefish	25	brewer's yeast		
6	Beech Family	48	bok choy	48	broccoli		

48	cabbage	17	cashew	66b	cherry	71	chufa
74	cacao	29	cassaba melon	6	chestnut	66a	cider, apple
12	Cactus Family	73	cassava	16	chevril	37	cinnamon
46	camote	37	cassia bark	45	chia seed	67	citron
31	cane sugar	73	castor bean	111	chicken	31	citronella
13	Canna Family	73	castor oil	38	chick-pea	67	Citrus Family
29	cantaloupe	118	catfish (ocean)	68	chicle	107	clam
14	caper	86	catfish species	18	chicory	45	clary
63	capsicum	45	catnip	63	chili pepper	49	clove
54	caramboia	48	cauliflower	48	Chinese cabbage	38	clover
16	caraway seed	125	caviar	22	Chinese	74	cocoa
26	cardamom	63	cayenne pepper		gooseberry	74	cocoa butter
18	cardoon	16	celeriac	80	Chinese potato	55	coconut
90	caribou	16	celery	29	Chinese	29	cocozelle
38	carob	18	celtuce		preserving melon	87	cod (scrod)
106	carp	4	ceriman	71	Chinese water	41	coffee
15	Carpetweed	18	chamomile		chestnut	74	cola nut
	Family	30	champagne	6	chinquapin	48	collards
1	carrageen	28	chard	39	chives	18	coltsfoot
16	carrot	29	chayote	74	chocolate	48	colza shoots
29	caserta squash	20	cherimoya	106	chub	9	comfrey

19	Conifer Family	31	couscous	89	crayfish	16	cumin
16	coriander	48	couve tronchuda	30	cream of tartar	48	curly cress
31	corn	38	cowpea	29	crenshaw melon	70	currant
77	corn-salad	89	crab	88	croaker	29	cushaw squash
18	costmary	66a	crabapple	29	crookneck	87	cusk
42	cottonseed oil	32	cranberry		squash	20	custard-apple
38	coumarin	126	crappie	29	cucumber		

D

95	dab	55	date sugar	22	Dillenia Family	30	dried currant
18	dandelion	90	deer	45	dittany	88	drum (saltwater)
4	dasheen	66c	dewberry	91	dolphin	93	duck
55	date	16	dill	92	dove	1	dulse

E

26	East Indian	63	eggplant	114	emu	18	escarole
	arrowroot	34	elderberry	18	endive	49	eucalyptus
23	Ebony Family	90	elk	79	English walnut		

F

38	fava bean	47	fig	16	finocchio	95	flounder
16	fennel	75	Fiji arrowroot	24	flaxseed	18	French endive
38	fenugreek	7	filbert	16	Florence fennel	96	frog
77	fetticus	37	file	21	Florida arrowroot	25	fungi

G

38	garbanzo	31	gluten flour	16	gotu kola	63	ground cherry
10	garden sorrel	85	goat	29	Gourd Family	71	groundnut
39	garlic	29	golden nugget	31	graham flour	117	grouper
39	garlic chives		squash	57	granadilla	97	grouse (ruffed)
29	gherkin	18	goldenrod	30	grape	49	guava
19	gin	11	golden seal	67	grapefruit	98	guinea fowl
26	ginger	93	goose	31	Grass Family	38	gum acacia
27	ginseng	70	gooseberry	61	grenadine		
18	globe artichoke	28	Goosefoot Family	31	grits		

H

87	haddock	47	hemp	29	honeydew	35	horsetail
87	hake	42	hibiscus	34	Honeysuckle	29	hubbard squash
95	halibut	79	hican		Family	32	huckleberry
100	harvest fish	79	hickory nut	47	hop	45	hyssop
7	hazelnut	127	hog	45	horehound		
79	heartnut	33	Holly Family	102	horse		
32	Heath Family	31	hominy	48	horseradish		

I

36	Iris Family	1	Irish Moss

J

23	Japanese persimmon	18	Jerusalem artichoke	38	jicama
				19	juniper

K

23	kaki	1	kelp	48	kohlrabi
48	kale	38	kidney bean	38	kudzu
31	kamut	22	kiwi berry	67	kumquat

L

85	lamb	67	lemon	39	Lily Family	66c	longberry
28	lamb's-quarters	45	lemon balm	38	lima bean	29	loofah
37	Laurel Family	31	lemon grass	67	lime	66a	loquat
45	lavender	78	lemon verbena	40	linden	16	lovage
38	lecithin	38	lentil	72	litchi	72	lychee
39	leek	18	lettuce	89	lobster		
38	Legume Family	38	licorice	66c	loganberry		

M

64	macadamia	44	Maple Family	25	morel	110	muskellunge
51	mace	45	marjoram	46	Morning-Glory	29	muskmelon
104	mackerel	105	marlin		Family	107	mussel
41	Madder Family	33	mate	25	mould	48	Mustard Family
4	malanga	101	menhaden	47	mulberry	48	mustard greens
42	Mallow Family	3	mescal	108	mullet	48	mustard seed
43	Malpighia Family	31	millet	38	mung bean	85	mutton
31	malt	45	Mint Family	67	murcot	49	Myrtle Family
31	maltose	31	molasses	30	muscadine		
17	mango	90	moose	25	mushroom		

N

80	name	38	navy bean	15	New Zealand	51	nutmeg
48	napa	66b	nectarine		spinach	25	nutritional yeast
50	nasturtium			112	northern scup		

O

31	oat	42	okra	53	Orchid Family	107	oyster
31	oatmeal	52	olive	45	oregano	18	oyster plant
118	ocean catfish	39	onion	36	orris root		
116	ocean perch	109	opossum	114	ostrich		
7	oil of birch	67	orange	54	oxalis		

P

48	pak choi (bok choy)	29	pattypan squash	63	pepino	65	pigweed
55	palm cabbage	20	pawpaw	63	pepper, sweet	110	pike
55	Palm Family	38	pea	59	peppercorn	101	pilchard (sardine)
56	papaya	66b	peach	29	Pepper Family	49	pimenta
63	paprika	111	peafowl	45	peppermint	63	pimiento
69	paradise nut	38	peanut	110	perch (yellow)	60	pineapple
16	parsley	66a	pear	29	Persian melon	19	pine nut
16	parsnip	79	pecan	23	persimmon	17	pistachio
97	partridge	66a	pectin	111	pheasant	95	plaice
57	passion fruit	58	Pedalium Family	110	pickerel	5	plantain
31	patent flour	45	pennyroyal	92	pigeon (squab)	66b	plum

4	poi	62	Poppy Family	29	preserving melon	67	pummelo
17	poison ivy	62	poppyseed	12	prickly pear	29	pumpkin
87	pollack	112	porgy	64	Protea Family	127	pumpkinseed (sunfish)
61	pomegranate	128	pork	66b	prune		
103	pompano	63	potato	25	puffball	65	Purslane Family
31	popcorn	89	prawn	3	pulque	18	pyrethrum

Q

111	quail	12	Queensland arrowroot	64	Queensland nut	2	quinoa
				66a	quince		

R

99	rabbit	38	red clover	101	roe	67	Rue Family
48	radish	122	red snapper	18	romaine	97	ruffed grouse
30	raisin	90	reindeer	66	Rose Family	48	rutabaga
39	ramp	10	rhubarb	116	rosefish	31	rye
48	rape	31	rice	66	rosehips		
66c	raspberry	85	Rocky Mountain sheep	42	roselle		
121	rattlesnake			45	rosemary		

S

18	safflower	70	Saxifrage Family	89	shrimp	45	spearmint
36	saffron	107	scallop	88	silver perch	31	spelt
45	sage	18	scolymus	119	silverside	28	spinach
55	sago starch	18	scorzonera	104	skipjack	88	spot
105	sailfish	117	Sea Bass Family	66b	sloe	88	spotted sea trout
115	salmon species	10	sea grape	120	smelt	73	Spurge Family
18	salsify	101	sea herring	107	snail	29	squash
18	santolina	88	sea trout	122	Snapper Family	107	squid
68	Sapodilla Family	1	seaweed	72	Soapberry Family	123	squirrel
69	Sapucaya Family	71	Sedge Family	39	soap plant	74	Sterculia Family
69	sapucaya nut	38	senna	95	sole	18	stevia
101	sardine	58	sesame	31	sorghum	66c	strawberry
39	sarsaparilla	101	shad	10	sorrel	38	string bean
37	sassafras	39	shallot	18	southernwood	124	sturgeon
110	sauger (perch)	35	shavegrass	38	soybean	126	sucker
45	savory	85	sheep	38	soy products	28	sugar beet

31	sugar cane	18	sunflower seed	31	sweet corn	128	swordfish
45	summer savory	48	swede	63	sweet pepper		
126	sunfish	16	sweet cicely	46	sweet potato		

T

75	Tacca Family	4	taro	129	tilefish	25	truffle
58	tahini	18	tarragon	63	tobacco	104	tuna
38	tamarind	66c	tayberry	63	tomatillo	29	turban squash
28	tampala	76	tea	63	tomato	95	turbot
67	tangelo	31	teff	38	tonka bean	130	turkey
67	tangerine	3	tequila	63	tree tomato	26	turmeric
18	tansy	131	terrapin	31	triticale	48	turnip
73	tapioca	45	thyme	115	trout species	132	turtle species

U

67	ugli fruit	48	upland cress

V

77	Valerian Family	85	veal	90	venison	66a	vinegar
53	vanilla	29	vegetable spaghetti	78	Verbena Family		(apple cider)

W

110	walleye	132	whale	59	white pepper	7	wintergreen
79	Walnut Family	31	wheat	110	white perch	45	winter savory
48	watercress	31	wheat germ	31	wild rice	18	witloof chicory
29	watermelon	119	whitebait	66c	wineberry	41	woodruff
88	weakfish	133	whitefish	30	wine vinegar	18	wormwood

Y

80	yam	4	yautia	110	yellow perch	73	yuca
80	yampi	82	yellow bass	33	yerba mate	39	yucca
18	yarrow	103	yellow jack	66c	youngberry		

Z

29	zucchini

Food Families

Numerical

1 Algae

agar agar
carrageen (irish moss)
dulse
kelp

2 Amaranth Family

amaranth
quinoa

3 Amaryllis Family

agave
mescal, pulque and tequila

4 Arum Family

ceriman
dasheen
malanga
taro
poi

5 Banana Family

arrowroot (Musa)
banana
plantain

6 Beech Family

chestnut
chinquapin

7 Birch Family

filbert (hazelnut)
oil of birch (winter green) (some winter-green flavour is methyl salicylate)

8 Bixa Family

annatto (natural yellow dye)

9 Borage Family

borage
comfrey (leaf & root)

10 Buckwheat Family

buckwheat
garden sorrel
rhubarb
sea grape

11 Buttercup Family

golden seal

12 Cactus Family

prickly pear

13 Canna Family

Queensland arrowroot

14 Caper Family

caper

15 Carpetweed Family

New Zealand spinach

16 Carrot Family

angelica
anise
caraway
carrot
celeriac (celery root)
celery (seed & leaf)
chevril
coriander
cumin
dill
   dill seed
fennel
   finocchio
   florence fennel
gotu kola
lovage
parsley
parsnip
sweet cicely

17 Cashew Family

cashew
mango
pistachio
poison ivy
poison oak
poison sumac

18 Composite Family

boneset
burdock root
cardoon
chamomile
chicory
coltsfoot
costmary
dandelion
endive
escarole
globe artichoke
Jerusalem artichoke
lettuce
   celtuce
pyrethrum
romaine
safflower oil
salsify (oyster plant)
santolina (herb)
scolymus (Spanish oyster plant)
scorzonera (black salsify)
southernwood
stevia
sunflower
sunflower seed, meal, oil
tansy (herb)
tarragon (herb)
witloof
wormwood (absinthe)
yarrow

19 Conifer Family

juniper (gin)
pine nut

20 Custard-Apple Family

cherimoya
custard-apple
pawpaw

21 Cycad Family

Florida arrowroot

22 Dillenia Family

Chinese gooseberry (kiwi berry)

23 Ebony Family

American persimmon
kaki (Japanese persimmon)

24 Flax Family

flaxseed

25 Fungi

baker's yeast
brewer's yeast
mould
   citric acid
morel
mushroom
puffball
truffle

26 Ginger Family

cardamom
East Indian arrowroot
ginger
turmeric

27 Ginseng Family

American ginseng
Chinese ginseng

28 Goosefoot Family

beet
chard
lamb's quarters
spinach
sugar beet
tampala

29 Gourd Family

chayote
Chinese melon
cucumber
gherkin
loofah (vegetable
sponge)
muskmelons
  cantaloupe
  casaba
  crenshaw
  honeydew
  Persian melon
pumpkin
  pumpkin seed
  & meal
squashes
  acorn
  buttercup
  butternut
  Boston marrow
  caserta

cocozelle
crookneck &
straighneck
cushaw
golden nugget
Hubbard varieties
pattypan
turban
spaghetti
zucchini
watermelon

30 Grape Family

grape
  brandy
  champagne
  cream of tartar
  dried currant
  raisin
  wine
  wine vinegar
muscadine

31 Grass Family

barley
  malt
  maltose
bamboo shoots
corn
  cornmeal
  corn oil
  cornstarch
  corn sugar
  corn syrup
  hominy grits
  popcorn
lemon grass
  citronella
millet

oat
  oatmeal
rice
  rice flour
rye
teff
sorghum
sugar cane
  cane sugar
  molasses
  raw sugar
sweet corn
triticale
wheat
  bran
  bulgar
  wheat germ
kamut
spelt
couscous

32 Heath Family

bearberry
blueberry
cranberry
huckleberry

33 Holly Family

mate (yerba mate)

34 Honeysuckle Family

eldeberry
  eldeberry flowers

35 Horsetail Family

shavegrass (horsetail)

36 Iris Family

orrisroot
saffron

37 Laurel Family

avocado
bay leaf
cassia bark
cinnamon
sassafras
  filé
  (powdered leaves)

38 Legume Family

alfalfa (sprouts)
beans
  fava
  lima
  mung (sprouts)
  navy
  string (kidney)
black-eyed pea
(cowpea)
carob
  carob syrup
chickpea (garbanzo)
fenugreek
gum acacia
gum tragacanth
jicama
kudzu
lentil
licorice
pea
peanut
  peanut oil
red clover
senna
soybean
  lecithin
  soy flour
  soy grits
  soy milk
  soy oil

tamarind
tonka bean
coumarin

39 Lily Family

aloe vera
asparagus
chives
garlic
garlic chives
leek
onion
ramp
sarsaparilla
shallot
yucca (soap plant)

40 Linden Family

basswood (linden)

41 Madder Family

coffee
woodruff

42 Mallow Family

althea root
cottonseed oil
hibiscus (roselle)
okra

43 Malpighia Family

acerola
(Barbados cherry)

44 Maple Family

maple sugar
maple syrup

45 Mint Family

apple mint
basil

bergamot
catnip
chia seed
clary
dittany
horehound
hyssop
lavender
lemon balm
marjoram
oregano
pennyroyal
peppermint
rosemary
sage
spearmint
summer savory
thyme
winter savory

46 Morning-Glory Family

camote
sweet potato

47 Mulberry Family

breadfruit
fig
hemp
hop
mulberry

48 Mustard Family

bok choy
broccoli
Brussels sprouts
cabbage
cardoon
cauliflower
Chinese cabbage
collards

colza shoots
couve tronchuda
curly cress
horseradish
kale
kohlrabi
mustard greens
mustard seed
napa
radish
rape
rutabaga
turnip
upland cress
watercress

49 Myrtle Family

allspice (pimenta)
clove
eucalyptus
guava

50 Nasturtium Family

nasturtium

51 Nutmeg Family

nutmeg
mace

52 Olive Family

olive
olive oil

53 Orchid Family

vanilla

54 Oxalis Family

carambola
oxalis

55 Palm Family

coconut
coconut meal
coconut oil
date
date sugar
palm cabbage
sago starch

56 Papaya Family

papaya

57 Passion Flower Family

granadilla
(passion fruit)

58 Pedalium Family

sesame seed
sesame oil
tahini

59 Pepper Family

peppercorn
black pepper
white pepper

60 Pineapple Family

pineapple

61 Pomegranate Family

pomegranate
grenadine

62 Poppy Family

poppyseed

63 Potato Family

eggplant
ground cherry

pepino (melon pear)
pepper (capsicum)
 bell, sweet
 cayenne
 chili
 paprika
 pimiento
potato
tobacco
tomatillo
tomato
tree tomato

64 Protea Family
macadamia
(Queensland nut)

65 Purslane Family
pigweed (purslane)

66 Rose Family
a) pomes
 apple
  cider
  vinegar
  pectin
 crabapple
 loquat
 pear
 quince
 rosehips
b) stone fruits
 almond
 apricot
 cherry
 peach (nectarine)
 plum (prune)
 sloe
c) berries
 blackberry
boysenberry
dewberry
loganberry
longberry
tayberry
youngberry
raspberry (leaf)
 black raspberry
 red raspberry
 purple raspberry
strawberry (leaf)
 wineberry
d) herb
 burnet
 (cucumber flavour)

67 Rue (citrus) Family
citron
grapefruit
kumquat
lemon
lime
murcot
orange
pummelo
tangelo
tangerine
ugli fruit

68 Sapodilla Family
chicle (chewing gum)

69 Sapucaya Family
Brazil nut
sapucaya nut
 (paradise nut)

70 Saxifrage Family
currant
gooseberry

71 Sedge Family
Chinese water
chestnut
chufa (groundnut)

72 Soapberry Family
litchi (lychee)

73 Spurge Family
cassava or yuca
 cassava meal
 tapioca (Brazilian arrowroot)
castor bean
 castor oil

74 Sterculia Family
chocolate (cacao)
cocoa
 cocoa butter
cola nut

75 Tacca Family
Fiji arrowroot

76 Tea Family
tea

77 Valerian Family
corn salad (fetticus)

78 Verbena Family
lemon verbena

79 Walnut Family
black walnut
butternut
English walnut
heartnut
hican
hickory nut
pecan

80 Yam Family
Chinese potato (yam)
name (yampi)

81 Anchovy Family
anchovy

82 Bass Family
yellow bass

83 Bear Family
bear

84 Bluefish Family
bluefish

85 Bovine Family
beef
beef by-products
gelatin
oleomargarine
rennin (rennet)
sausage casings
suet
milk products
 butter
 cheese
 ice cream
 lactose
 spray-dried milk
 yogurt
veal
buffalo (bison)
goat
 cheese
 ice cream
 milk

sheep
  lamb
  mutton
  rocky mountain

86 Catfish Family

catfish

87 Codfish Family

cod (scrod)
cusk
haddock
hake
pollack

88 Croaker Family

croaker
drum
sea troout
silver perch
spot
spotted sea trout

89 Crustaceans

crab
crayfish
lobster
prawn
shrimp

90 Deer Family

caribou
deer (venison)
elk
moose
reindeer

91 Dolphin Family

dolphin

92 Dove Family

dove
pigeon (squab)

93 Duck Family

duck eggs
goose eggs

94 Eel Family

American eel

95 Flounder Family

dab
flounder
halibut
plaice
sole
turbot

96 Frog Family

frog

97 Grouse Family

ruffed grouse
(partridge)

98 Guinea Fowl Family

guinea fowl eggs

99 Hare Family

rabbit

100 Harvestfish Family

butterfish
harvestfish

101 Herring Family

menhaden
pilchard
sea herring
shad
sprat
sardine

102 Horse Family

horse

103 Jack Family

amberjack
pompano
yellow jack

104 Mackerel Family

albacore
bonito
mackerel
skipjack
tuna

105 Marlin Family

marlin
sailfish

106 Minnow

carp
chub

107 Mollusks

Gastropods
  abalone
  snail
Cephalopods
  squid
Pelecypods
  clam
  cockle
  mussel
  oyster
  scallop

108 Mullet Family

mullet

109 Opossum Family

opossum

110 Perch and Pike Family

muskellunge
pickerel
pike
sauger
walleye
yellow perch

111 Pheasant Family

chicken eggs
peafowl
pheasant
quail

112 Porgy Family

northern scup
(porgy)

113 Pronghorn Family

antelope

114 Ratite Family

emu
ostrich
rhea

115 Salmon Family

salmon
trout

116 Scorpionfish Family

rosefish (ocean perch)

117 Sea Bass Family
grouper
sea bass

118 Sea Catfish Family
ocean catfish

119 Silverside Family
silverside (whitebait)

120 Smelt Family
smelt

121 Snake Family
rattlesnake

122 Snapper Family
red snapper

123 Squirrel Family
squirrel

124 Sturgeon Family
sturgeon (caviar)

125 Sucker Family
buffalowfish
sucker

126 Sunfish Family
black bass species
sunfish species
  pumpkinseed
crappie

127 Swine Family
hog (pork)
  bacon
  ham
  lard
  pork gelatin
  sausage
  scrapple

128 Swordfish Family
swordfish

129 Tilefish Family
tilefish

130 Turkey Family
turkey eggs

131 Turtle Family
terrapin
turtle species

132 Whale Family
whale

133 Whitefish Family
whitefish

Sample Rotation Diet

Day 1

Protein
- 85 beef, buffalo, beef gelatin, veal, lamb, mutton, goat
- 90 moose, deer, caribou

Vegetables
- 63 potato, tomato, eggplant, garden/hot pepper
- 25 mushrooms
- 52 olive
- 5 plantain
- 4 dasheen (white yam)

Fruits
- 66 strawberry, raspberry, blackberry, boysenberry, apple, pear, quince, apricot, cherry, nectarine, peach, plum, prune
- 37 avocado
- 12 prickly pear
- 5 banana
- 63 ground cherry

Spices
- 37 sassafras, bay leaf, cinnamon
- 36 saffron
- 59 black, white pepper
- 63 pepper— chili, paprika, cayenne, pimiento
- 66 rosehips

Grains
- 31 millet, corn, spelt, oats, wheat, rye, barley, rice, wild rice, teff, kamut
- 63 potato starch or flour
- 4, 5, 21 arrowroot flour

Oils
- 85 butter
- 52 olive oil
- 24 flaxseed oil
- 66 almond oil, butter

Nuts and Seeds
- 66 almond
- 19 pine nut
- 24 flax

Drinks
- 66 apple juice, pear juice
- 37 sassafras tea
- 85 cow's milk, goat's milk
- 63 tomato juice
- 31 rice milk

Sweeteners
- 31 rice syrup, barley malt, barley sugar, corn syrup

Day 2

Protein			Grains		
	114	emu, ostrich		73	cassava, tapioca
	130	turkey			
	111	chicken, cornish hen, quail eggs	Oils	73	castor oil
	99	rabbit		29	pumpkin seed oil
	93	duck, goose			

Vegetables			Nuts and Seeds		
	29	cucumber, squash, pumpkin, zucchini		69	brazil nuts
	39	asparagus, leek, chive, onion, garlic, shallot		29	pumpkin seed
				62	poppy seed
				47	hemp nut

Fruits			Drinks		
	29	cantaloupe, watermelon, all other melons		32	cranberry juice
	32	blueberry, cranberry, huckleberry		39	aloe vera juice

Sweeteners		
	47	fig syrup

Spices		
	39	garlic, chive
	53	vanilla (orchid family)
	51	mace, nutmeg
	26	cardamom, ginger, turmeric
	11	goldenseal

Day 3

Protein		
87	cod, haddock, pollack	
110	perch, walleye	
104	tuna, mackerel	
95	halibut, flounder, sole, turbot	
84	bluefish	

Vegetables
- 38 alfalfa, peas, beans, lentils, soybeans
- 16 parsley, carrot, celery, celeriac, parsnip, fennel
- 71 water chestnuts

Fruits
- 55 dates, coconut, sago
- 70 currants, gooseberry
- 67 lemon, lime, grapefruit, tangelo, all oranges, kumquat
- 17 mango
- 56 papaya

Spices
- 9 comfrey, senna, coumarin, fenugreek
- 38 licorice, carob, anise, caraway, celery seed, dill, coriander, cumin, parsley, fennel

Grains
- 38 soy flour, carob flour, bean, pea flour, chickpea flour, gum acacia

Oils
- 38 soy oil, peanut oil, lecithin
- 9 borage
- 55 coconut oil

Nuts and Seeds
- 38 peanut, soy nut
- 6 chestnut
- 17 pistachio, cashew
- 64 macadamia

Drinks
- 56 papaya juice
- 38 soy milk
- 67 orange, lemon, grapefruit
- 35 horsetail tea

Sweeteners
- 55 date sugar

Day 4

Protein		
	132	turtle
	127	pork
	107	abalone, clam, snail, squid, mussel, scallop, oyster

Vegetables		
	48	cabbage, kale, broccoli, brussels sprouts, radish, kohlrabi, turnip, cauliflower, mustard greens, watercress
	80	yam
	46	sweet potato
	10	sorrel

Fruits		
	30	grapes, raisins
	60	pineapple
	10	rhubarb
	61	pomegranate
	22	kiwi

Spices		
	48	horseradish, mustard
	30	cream of tartar
	45	basil, oregano, mint, sage, thyme, rosemary, marjoram, catnip, bergamot, lavender

Grains		
	10	buckwheat, (every 10 days only)

Oils		
	79	walnut oil
	127	lard (pork)

Nuts and Seeds		
	79	walnut, pecan, butternut, hickory, black walnut

Drinks		
	30	grape juice
	60	pineapple juice
	45	mint tea
	74	cocoa, cola nut

Sweeteners		
	30	grape juice
	44	maple sugar, maple syrup

Day 5

Protein			Grains		
	117	grouper, sea bass		2	amaranth, quinoa
	115	salmon, trout		18	Jerusalem artichoke flour
	134	whitefish			
	81	anchovy	Oils	58	sesame oil
	89	crab, lobster, shrimp		18	sunflower oil, safflower oil
	118	ocean catfish		42	cottonseed oil
	120	smelt			

Protein
- 117 grouper, sea bass
- 115 salmon, trout
- 134 whitefish
- 81 anchovy
- 89 crab, lobster, shrimp
- 118 ocean catfish
- 120 smelt

Vegetables
- 28 sugar beet, spinach, beets, swiss chard
- 18 artichoke, endive, lettuce, chicory, romaine
- 42 okra
- 28 lamb's quarters

Fruits
- 49 guava
- 47 mulberry, figs
- 72 lychee nut

Spices
- 49 eucalyptus, allspice, cloves, guava
- 14 capers
- 18 burdock root, camomile, dandelion, tarragon

Grains
- 2 amaranth, quinoa
- 18 Jerusalem artichoke flour

Oils
- 58 sesame oil
- 18 sunflower oil, safflower oil
- 42 cottonseed oil

Nuts and Seeds
- 7 filbert, hazelnut
- 58 sesame seed, tahini
- 18 sunflower seed

Drinks
- 18 chamomile, chicory tea
- 7 wintergreen

Sweeteners
- 28 beet sugar
- 18 stevia

Allergen Avoidance
Index

Legend

WF: wheat free

YF: yeast free

DF: dairy free

EF: egg free

CF: corn free

RSF: refined sugar free

SF: soy free

NF: nut free

GF: gluten free

* can be omitted

		WF	YF	DF	EF	CF	RSF	SF	NF	GF
48	Muesli	X	X	X	X	X	X	X		X
49	Maple Granola	X	X	X	X	X	X	X	X*	X
50	Rice Porridge	X	X	X	X	X	X	X	X*	X
51	Banana Oatmeal	X	X	X	X	X	X	X	X	X
52	Hot Cereal	X	X	X	X	X	X	X	X*	X*
53	Fig Butter	X	X	X	X	X	X	X	X	X
54	Spelt Pancakes	X	X	X	X	X	X	X*	X	
55	Blueberry Buckwheat Pancakes	X	X	X	X	X	X	X	X	X
56	Quinoa Pancakes	X	X	X	X	X	X	X	X	X
57	Yummy Teff Pancakes	X	X	X	X	X	X	X	X	X
58	Millet Applejacks	X	X	X	X	X	X	X	X	X
59	Morning Quinoa	X	X	X	X	X	X	X	X*	X
60	Scrambled Tofu	X	X	X	X	X	X	X	X	X
61	Applesauce Breakfast Cake	X	X	X	X	X	X	X		X*
62	Squash Cranberry Muffins	X	X	X	X	X	X	X	X	X*

	WF	YF	DF	EF	CF	RSF	SF	NF	GF
63 Juice for Candida	X	X	X	X	X	X	X	X	X
63 Juice for increasing Potassium	X	X	X	X	X	X	X	X	X
63 Cleansing Juice	X	X	X	X	X	X	X	X	X
63 Calcium-Rich Juice	X	X	X	X	X	X	X	X	X

Main Dishes and Lunches

	WF	YF	DF	EF	CF	RSF	SF	NF	GF
66 Walnut Burgers	X	X*	X	X	X	X	X		
67 Hemp Burgers	X	X*	X	X	X	X	X	X	
68 Bean and Rice Burgers	X	X*	X	X	X	X	X	X	
69 Filling for Spelt Wraps	X*	X	X	X	X	X	X	X	
70 Rice Roll Ups	X	X	X	X	X	X	X	X	X
71 Almond Gravy	X	X	X	X	X	X	X		X
72 Salmon Croquettes	X	X*	X	X	X	X	X	X	
73 Ratatouille	X	X	X	X	X	X	X	X	X
74 Vegetarian Shepherd's Pie	X	X	X	X	X	X	X	X	X

		WF	YF	DF	EF	CF	RSF	SF	NF	GF
76	Beef Shepherd's Pie	X	X	X	X	X*	X	X	X	X
77	Lentil Shepherd's Pie	X	X	X	X	X	X	X	X	X
78	Baked Beans	X	X	X	X	X	X	X	X	X
80	Easy Beef or Lamb Stew	X	X	X	X	X*	X	X	X*	X*
82	Stuffed Lamb	X	X	X	X	X	X	X	X	X*
83	Pineapple Meatballs	X	X	X	X	X*	X		X	X
84	Caribou Meatloaf	X	X	X	X	X	X	X	X	X
85	Chutney	X	X	X	X	X	X	X	X	X
86	Beef Stir Fry	X	X	X	X	X	X	X	X	X
88	Stuffed Grape Leaves	X	X	X	X	X	X	X	X	X
89	Tuna and Pasta	X	X	X	X	X	X	X	X	X*
90	Sweet and Sour Chicken	X	X	X	X	X	X	X	X	X
91	Simple Chicken Dinner	X	X	X	X	X	X	X	X	X
92	Garlic Shrimp with Lime	X	X	X	X	X	X	X	X	X
93	Barbequed Red Snapper	X	X	X	X	X	X	X	X	X
94	BBQ Fish Fillet	X	X	X	X	X	X	X	X	X
95	Fish Fingers	X	X	X	X	X	X	X*	X*	X*
96	Vegetarian Tourtière	X	X	X	X	X	X	X	X	

		WF	YF	DF	EF	CF	RSF	SF	NF	GF
101	Red Lentil and Sweet Potato	X	X	X	X	X	X	X	X	X
102	Parsnip	X	X	X	X	X	X	X	X	X
103	Millet Vegetable	X	X	X	X	X	X	X	X	X
104	Creamy Cauliflower	X	X	X	X	X	X	X	X	X
105	Carrot	X	X	X	X	X	X	X	X	X
106	Leek and Potato	X	X	X	X	X	X	X	X	X
107	Split Pea	X	X	X	X	X	X	X	X	X
108	Veggie Barley	X	X	X	X	X	X	X	X	
109	Spinach and Pear	X	X	X	X	X	X	X	X	X
110	Cream of Broccoli	X	X	X	X	X	X	X	X	X
111	Quinoa	X	X	X	X	X	X	X	X	X
112	Zucchini	X	X	X	X	X	X	X	X	X
113	Bortsch	X	X	X	X	X	X	X	X	X

		WF	YF	DF	EF	CF	RSF	SF	NF	GF
116	Quinoa Salad	X	X	X	X	X	X	X	X	X
117	Sweet Potato Salad	X	X	X	X	X	X	X	X	X
118	Potato Salad	X	X	X	X	X	X		X	X
119	Fruit Salad	X	X	X	X	X	X	X	X	X
120	Good Ol'Fashioned Cabbage Salad	X	X	X	X	X	X		X	X
121	Waldorf Salad	X	X	X	X	X	X			X
122	Buckwheat Noodle Salad	X	X	X	X	X	X	X	X	X
123	Lentil Salad with Cucumber and Fennel	X	X	X	X	X	X	X	X	X
124	Asparagus and Shrimp Salad	X	X	X	X	X	X	X	X	X
125	Rice Salad	X	X	X	X	X	X	X	X	X
126	Rice, Lentil and Olive Salad	X	X	X	X	X	X	X	X	X
127	Caesar Salad	X	X	X	X	X	X		X	X
128	Mung Bean Noodle Salad	X	X	X	X	X	X		X	X
129	Cauliflower and Broccoli Salad	X	X	X	X	X	X	X	X	X

		WF	YF	DF	EF	CF	RSF	SF	NF	GF
130	My Favourite Herb Dressing	X	X	X	X	X	X	X	X	X
131	Sunflower Dressing	X	X	X	X	X	X	X	X	X
132	French Dressing	X	X	X	X	X	X	X	X	X
133	Simple Olive Oil Dressing	X	X	X	X	X	X	X	X	X
134	Italian Dressing	X	X	X	X	X	X	X	X	X
135	Thai Dressing	X	X	X	X	X	X	X	X	X
136	Basil and Red Pepper Dressing	X	X	X	X	X	X	X	X	X
137	Dairy-Free Caesar Dressing	X	X	X	X	X	X		X	X
138	Soyannaise	X	X	X	X	X	X		X	X
139	Creamy Cucumber Dressing	X	X	X	X	X	X			X
140	Pesto	X	X	X	X	X	X	X		X
141	Vegetable Stuffing	X	X	X	X	X	X	X	X	
142	Beef Marinade	X	X	X	X	X	X	X	X	X
143	Chicken Marinade	X	X	X	X	X	X		X	X
144	Lamb Marinade	X	X	X	X	X	X		X	X
145	Chicken Salsa	X	X	X	X	X	X	X	X	X

		WF	YF	DF	EF	CF	RSF	SF	NF	GF
148	Yummy Red Lentil Dip	X	X	X	X	X	X	X	X	X
149	Sesame Crackers	X	X	X	X	X	X	X	X	X*
150	Crispies	X	X	X	X	X	X	X		X
151	Good Ol' Hummus	X	X	X	X	X	X	X	X	X
152	Sweet Potato Pâté	X	X	X	X	X	X	X	X	X
154	Vegetarian Pâté	X	X	X	X	X	X	X	X	X*
155	Carrot Loaf	X	X	X	X*	X	X	X		X
156	Nibble Mix	X	X	X	X	X	X	X	X*	X
157	Homemade Fries	X	X	X	X	X	X	X	X	X
158	Garbanzo Spread	X	X	X	X	X	X	X	X	X
159	Parsnip Spread	X	X	X	X	X	X			X
160	Eggplant Dip or Pasta Sauce	X	X	X	X	X	X	X	X	X
161	Tofu Spread	X	X	X	X	X	X		X	X
162	White Bean Dip	X	X	X	X	X	X	X	X	X
163	Pizza	X	X	X	X	X	X	X	X	X

		WF	YF	DF	EF	CF	RSF	SF	NF	GF
166	Mum's Homemade Apple Sauce	X	X	X	X	X	X	X	X	X
167	Apple Pudding	X	X	X	X	X	X	X	X	X
168	Blueberry Muffins	X	X	X	X	X	X	X	X	
169	Banana Muffins	X	X	X	X	X	X	X	X	
170	Blueberry Banana Muffins	X	X	X	X	X	X	X	X	X
171	Apple Walnut Muffins	X	X	X	X	X	X	X		X
172	Peanut Butter Banana Muffins	X	X	X	X	X	X	X		X
173	Sweet Potato Dessert	X	X	X	X	X	X	X		X
174	Lemon Almond Biscotti	X	X	X	X	X	X	X		
176	Banana Date Cookies	X	X	X	X	X	X	X	X*	
177	Fruit and Nut Bars	X	X	X	X	X	X	X		X
178	Gingerbread Cookies	X	X	X	X	X	X	X		
179	Birthday Cake	X	X	X	X	X	X	X	X	X*
180	Pseudo-Brownies	X	X	X	X	X	X	X		X
181	Pseudo-Brownie Icing	X	X	X	X	X	X	X		X

	WF	YF	DF	EF	CF	RSF	SF	NF	GF
182 Date and Carob Icing	X	X	X	X	X	X	X	X	X
183 Carob Tahini Icing	X	X	X	X	X	X	X*	X*	X
184 Carrot Date Muffins	X	X	X	X	X	X	X	X	
185 Cranberry Loaf	X	X	X	X*	X	X	X	X	X*
186 Sweet Potato Muffins	X	X	X	X	X	X	X		X
187 Fruit Mousse	X	X	X	X	X	X	X*	X*	X
188 Carob Banana Pie	X	X	X	X	X	X	X		X
189 Sunflower Oat Bars	X	X	X	X	X	X	X	X	
190 Apple Crisp	X	X	X	X	X	X	X	X	X*
191 Strawberry Hemp Ice	X	X	X	X	X	X	X	X	X
192 Carob Banana Hemp Ice	X	X	X	X	X	X	X	X	X
193 Oatmeal Cookies	X	X	X	X	X	X	X	X	X*
194 Lime Coconut Cookies	X	X	X	X	X	X	X	X*	X
195 Christmas Treats	X	X	X	X	X	X	X		X
196 Christmas Cashew Balls	X	X	X	X	X	X	X		X
197 Orange Teff Cookies	X	X	X	X	X	X	X		X
198 Teff Peanut Butter Cookies	X	X	X	X	X	X	X		X

		WF	YF	DF	EF	CF	RSF	SF	NF	GF
199	Rice Pudding With Lemon	X	X	X	X	X	X	X	X	X
200	Barley Pudding	X	X	X	X	X	X	X	X	
201	Carrot Haystacks	X	X	X	X	X	X	X	X	X
202	Carob Haystacks	X	X	X	X	X	X	X	X	X
203	Cashew Muffins	X	X	X	X	X	X	X		

Metric Conversion

Canadian Metric	Conventional Measure
1 ml	1/4 teaspoon
2 ml	1/2 teaspoon
5 ml	1 teaspoon
10 ml	2 teaspoons
15 ml	1 tablespoon
30 ml	2 tablespoons
45 ml	3 tablespoons
50 ml	1/4 cup
75 ml	1/3 cup
125 ml	1/2 cup
150 ml	2/3 cup
175 ml	3/4 cup
250 ml	1 cup

About the Author

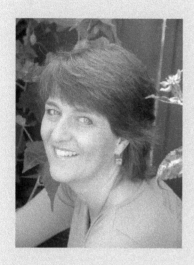

Shirley Plant has studied in the field of nutrition for many years. Diagnosed with chronic fatigue syndrome, fibromyalgia, and multiple food and environmental allergies, Shirley understands firsthand the difficulties of trying to plan creative, nutritious, and affordable menus while having to avoid such common foods as wheat, dairy, eggs, corn, gluten, and sugar, just to name a few. But through understanding, education, and a keen interest to help people find food alternatives to fit into their life schedules, Shirley has developed an expertise and reputation in dietary design, customized recipes, and menu-planning. For more information, please visit *www.deliciousalternatives.com*.

Lightning Source UK Ltd.
Milton Keynes UK
UKHW030634260719
346818UK00004B/189/P